D1742333

Multiple Choice Questions in General Pathology

Multiple Choice Questions in General Pathology

F. G. SMIDDY, MD, CHM, FRCS

Consultant Surgeon, General Infirmary, Leeds and Clayton Hospital, Wakefield. Senior Clinical Lecturer in Surgery, University of Leeds. Member of the Court of Examiners, the Royal College of Surgeons of England. Examiner in Pathology, Royal College of Surgeons of England

J. L. TURK, MD, DSC(LOND), FRCP, FRCS, FRCPATH

Sir William Collins Professor of Human and Comparative Pathology, the Royal College of Surgeons of England and the University of London. Examiner in Pathology, Royal College of Surgeons of England

Pitman

PITMAN BOOKS LIMITED
39 Parker Street, London WC2B 5PB

PITMAN PUBLISHING INC.
1020 Plain Street, Marshfield, Massachusetts

Associated Companies
Pitman Publishing Pty Ltd, Melbourne
Pitman Publishing New Zealand Ltd, Wellington
Copp Clark Pitman, Toronto

First Published 1981

British Library Cataloguing in Publication Data
Smiddy, F. G.
    Multiple choice questions in general pathology.
    1. Pathology – Miscellanea
    I. Title   II. Turk, J. L.
    616.07'76   RB119

ISBN: 0-272-79631-X

Text set in 9 on 11 pt Linotron 202 Palatino,
printed and bound in Great Britain
at The Pitman Press, Bath

Contents

Foreword

In all the Primary Examinations for the various Colleges of Surgery throughout the United Kingdom, Ireland and the Commonwealth the ability to answer a multiple choice question paper is now an important part of the examination. Indeed in some Colleges, the candidate who is unable to deal with this type of question is eliminated without further examination.

The object of this text book is twofold. Firstly a number of prospective candidates for one of the first part examinations may desire to test both their knowledge and technique. They may also wish to time themselves against the clock in order to ascertain that their 'work rate' is satisfactory. In order to achieve this object approximately 300 questions governing the principles of general pathology have been arranged in groups of 20 in a random fashion. Secondly a candidate may wish not only to practise the technique of answering the multiple choice question paper but also to add to his knowledge. For this latter reason in the second part of the book, each answer, whether it be true or false, is accompanied by explanation.

The stimulus to write this book comes from our many years of examining candidates in General Pathology. Although it would be incorrect to suggest that this text is a substitute for a normal text book, by dividing the questions into a variety of important topics we have done our best to achieve a comprehensive cover of the subjects as a whole.

F. G. SMIDDY

JULY 1981 J. TURK

Preface

The Authors of this book have stimulated to compose its contents following our contact with innumerable candidates in the Primary Fellowship over the past six years. We have attempted to cover the broad outlines of principles of general pathology by dividing the book into a number of different sections. Those candidates who wish to use the book merely for self-assessment will find that the questions in the first part of the book have been arranged in random fashion and, although the answers are given, no explanation as to the reason why the answer is true or false has been indicated in this section.

In the second section of the book the questions are repeated together with the answers and the explanation of the correct answer has been given in some detail so that the candidate who is wishing to learn rather than merely to test his own ability is able to do so.

We hope that this book will be found helpful by the many candidates who face the hurdle of the Primary Fellowships.

Acknowledgements

It is with deep gratitude that the Authors acknowledge the great help given to them by Margaret Smith and Lynn Topham, our respective secretaries, who dealt with many aspects of the unfinished manuscript. It would also be impossible to ignore the unflagging labours of Mrs P. Docherty who was responsible for the major typographical work on the written manuscript. It would also be right and proper to acknowledge the stimulus which the examination of numerous candidates in the Primary Fellowship of Pathology gave us.

F. G. SMIDDY
J. TURK

Part 1: Random questions

Each group of 20 questions is followed by the answers.

16.6 Liquefaction associated with necrosis occurs after infarction of the:

1. heart
2. kidney
3. brain
4. liver
5. spleen

7.24 Cell mediated immunity involves the following mechanisms:

1. IgG
2. T-lymphocytes
3. Eosinophil leucocytes
4. Complement
5. Macrophages

16.1 The chief pathological changes of atherosclerosis are:

1. deposition of lipid in the smooth muscle cells of the intima
2. fragmentation of the internal elastic lamina
3. calcification
4. contraction of the vessel
5. collagen deposition

10.3 Pulmonary oedema may occur in patients suffering from:

1. head injuries
2. plague
3. right-sided heart failure
4. hypoproteinaemia
5. nematode infections

1.3 Old age is specifically associated with atrophic changes in:

1. bone
2. the kidneys
3. the bone marrow
4. the brain
5. the ovaries

14.14 The following tumours may produce hormones

1. Choriocarcinoma
2. Bronchial carcinoma
3. Fibroma of the ovary
4. Islet cell tumours of the pancreas
5. Chromophobe pituitary adenoma

16.4 Gangrene is necrosis together with

1. desiccation
2. colliquative necrosis
3. involvement of a limb
4. infection of the tissues with Gram-positive organisms
5. putrefaction

20.8 Hyperkalaemia commonly occurs

1. following severe burns
2. in Conn's syndrome
3. following glomerular necrosis
4. in the Zollinger–Ellison syndrome
5. in the carcinoid syndrome

21.1 Blood which is to be used for transfusion:

1. should be stored at −4°C
2. may need to be irradiated (1000r)
3. needs to be tested for complement content
4. may be used after storage for platelet replacement
5. should be stored in an acid anticoagulant

3.5 Hyperplasia of the lymphoid tissue is a prominent feature in the following conditions:

1. Toxoplasmosis
2. Leishmaniasis
3. Chronic dermatitis
4. Silicosis
5. Berylliosis

4.7 Pseudomembranous enterocolitis is caused by the following organisms:

1. *Clostridium sporogenes*
2. *Clostridium difficile*
3. *Streptococcus faecalis*
4. Penicillin resistant staphylococci
5. *Pseudomonas aeruginosa*

4.5 The virulence of bacteria is related to:

1. their number in the tissues
2. the production of toxins
3. their ability to produce spreading factors
4. their resistance to phagocytosis
5. decreased resistance of the host

23.7 The following are mainly intracellular parasites:

1. *Echinococcus granulosus*
2. *Leishmania donovani*
3. *Trypanosoma gambiense*
4. *Plasmodium vivax*
5. *Toxoplasma gondii*

3.11 The following metals cause epithelioid cell granulomas:

1. Beryllium
2. Chromium
3. Zirconium
4. Nickel
5. Iron

6.2 Primary union of a wound is associated with the following:

1. A lag phase
2. A demolition phase
3. A contractile phase
4. A proliferative phase
5. A maturation phase

17.18 Chronic myeloid leukaemia is associated with:

1. the presence of large numbers of myeloblasts in the peripheral blood
2. a very variable total white count
3. massive splenomegaly
4. lymph node enlargement
5. hepatomegaly

18.7 The plasma acid phosphatase concentration increases in:

1. Paget's disease (osteitis deformans)
2. idiopathic hypercalciuria
3. prostatic cancer
4. medullary carcinoma of the thyroid
5. rickets

7.16 Anaphylaxis:

1. develops 24 hours after the initial stimulus
2. causes an urticarial eruption
3. is produced by IgA antibody
4. causes eosinophilia
5. causes degranulation of basophils and mast cells

7.33 Graft versus host disease:

1. may follow bone marrow transplants
2. may follow blood transfusion
3. occurs in Hodgkin's disease
4. can be suppressed by tetracyclines
5. can be suppressed by cyclophosphamide

6.1 Wound healing is enhanced by the administration of:

1. cortisol
2. zinc
3. aldosterone
4. oxygen
5. vitamin C

Answer

Question number	Answer				
16.6	1. F	2. F	3. T	4. F	5. F
7.24	1. F	2. T	3. F	4. F	5. T
16.1	1. T	2. T	3. T	4. F	5. T
10.3	1. T	2. T	3. F	4. F	5. F
1.3	1. T	2. T	3. T	4. T	5. T
14.14	1. T	2. T	3. F	4. T	5. T
16.4	1. F	2. F	3. F	4. F	5. T
20.8	1. T	2. F	3. T	4. F	5. F
21.1	1. F	2. T	3. F	4. F	5. T
3.5	1. T	2. F	3. T	4. F	5. F
4.7	1. F	2. T	3. F	4. T	5. F
4.5	1. F	2. T	3. T	4. T	5. F
23.7	1. F	2. T	3. F	4. T	5. T
3.11	1. T	2. F	3. T	4. F	5. F
6.2	1. T	2. T	3. F	4. T	5. T
17.18	1. F	2. T	3. T	4. F	5. T
18.7	1. F	2. F	3. T	4. F	5. F
7.16	1. F	2. T	3. F	4. T	5. T
7.33	1. T	2. T	3. F	4. F	5. T
6.1	1. F	2. T	3. F	4. T	5. T

12.11 The following coagulation factors are generated in the liver:

1. Factor II
2. Factor IV
3. Factor VI
4. Factor IX
5. Factor X

16.5 Infarction may occur as a complication in the following diseases:

1. Atherosclerosis
2. Monckeberg's sclerosis
3. Benign hypertension
4. Sickle-cell anaemia
5. Idiopathic thrombocytopenic purpura

10.4 Amyloid is deposited most frequently in:

1. liver
2. brain
3. spleen
4. lungs
5. kidneys

7.14 Immune complex disease may be associated with:

1. hepatitis B infection
2. skin graft rejection
3. Henoch–Schönlein disease
4. meningococcal infection
5. penicillin therapy

18.4 Primary thyrotoxicosis is always accompanied by:

1. increased iodine uptake by the gland
2. a raised protein bound iodine
3. exophthalmos
4. hypercalcaemia
5. pernicious anaemia

7.3 Bence–Jones proteins are:

1. the heavy chains of immunoglobulins
2. found in the urine in multiple myeloma
3. associated with a monoclonal gammopathy
4. found in the urine in Waldenström's macroglobu-linaemia
5. precipitated by boiling

7.30 Which of the following tests may be used to assess host resistance to mycobacterial infections:

1. Skin tests
2. Complement fixation
3. Lymphocyte transformation test
4. Radio immuno-assay
5. Leucocyte migration inhibition test

12.2 Haemolytic jaundice is associated with:

1. an increase in the concentration of bilirubin diglu-curonide in the bile
2. the presence of bilirubin in the urine
3. an increase in the serum alkaline phosphatase
4. a decrease in unconjugated bilirubin in the serum
5. an increase in urobilinogen in the urine

7.1 The following substances normally act as antigens, i.e. stimulate antibody production, when administered to humans:

1. Dextrans with a molecular weight below 150 000
2. Bovine insulin
3. Extracts of Primula
4. Human thyroglobulin
5. Rh.D antigen

12.8 Gall stones are associated with the following diseases:

1. Viral hepatitis
2. Cirrhosis of the liver
3. Haemolytic jaundice
4. Obesity
5. Raised serum triglycerides

22.4 The following are immunosuppressive drugs:

1. Azathioprine
2. Indomethacin
3. Oxyprenolol
4. Cyclophosphamide
5. Chlorpropamide

23.2 The 'sick cell syndrome' is associated with:

1. cardiac failure following surgery or trauma
2. failure of the sodium pump
3. a rise in the urinary sodium excretion
4. apathy
5. intracellular oedema

17.14 The following biochemical changes occur in pernicious anaemia:

1. A raised serum vitamin B_{12}
2. A normal serum folate
3. A raised serum bilirubin
4. An increased alkaline phosphatase
5. A decreased plasma copper

5.8 Antibiotics which inhibit the synthesis of mucopeptide in the wall of a bacterium include:

1. cycloserine
2. cephalosporins
3. neomycin
4. penicillin and its semisynthetic derivatives
5. erythromycin

10.7 The essential constituents of amyloid include:

1. immunoglobulins
2. complement
3. albumin
4. starch
5. fibrils

6.8 Woven bone is found:

1. in bone forming in a model of cartilage
2. in fracture haematomas
3. in bones forming in sheets of differentiating mesenchyme
4. replacing lamellar bone in healing fractures
5. surrounding the ends of ununited fractures

20.7 The metabolic effects following a severe injury include:

1. respiratory alkalosis
2. accelerated gluconeogenesis
3. mobilisation of fat stores
4. decreased aldosterone secretion
5. protein anabolism

17.7 The commonest haemolytic disorder in the world is:

1. congenital spherocytosis
2. disseminated lupus erythematosus
3. malaria
4. G6PD deficiency
5. sickle cell disease

2.12 Micro-organisms which have undergone phagocytosis are killed by:

1. lecithinase
2. lysozyme
3. lysosomal enzymes
4. lymphokine
5. hydrogen peroxide

5.1 When using an autoclave to sterilise surgical drapes and instruments it is essential that:

1. the load should be tightly packed
2. the containers in which the loads are packed should be impervious to steam
3. air should be completely removed from the chamber prior to the admission of steam
4. a vacuum must be made at the end of the cycle
5. an adequate indication of autoclave efficiency should be included in the load

Question number			Answer		
12.11	1. T	2. F	3. F	4. T	5. T
16.5	1. T	2. F	3. F	4. T	5. F
10.4	1. T	2. F	3. T	4. F	5. T
7.14	1. T	2. F	3. T	4. T	5. T
18.4	1. T	2. T	3. F	4. T	5. F
7.3	1. F	2. T	3. T	4. F	5. F
7.30	1. T	2. F	3. T	4. F	5. T
12.2	1. T	2. F	3. F	4. F	5. T
7.1	1. F	2. T	3. F	4. F	5. T
12.8	1. F	2. F	3. T	4. T	5. T
22.4	1. T	2. F	3. F	4. T	5. F
23.2	1. T	2. T	3. F	4. T	5. T
17.14	1. F	2. T	3. T	4. F	5. F
5.8	1. T	2. T	3. F	4. T	5. F
10.7	1. T	2. F	3. F	4. F	5. T
6.8	1. F	2. T	3. F	4. F	5. F
20.7	1. T	2. T	3. T	4. F	5. F
17.7	1. F	2. F	3. T	4. F	5. F
2.12	1. F	2. T	3. T	4. F	5. T
5.1	1. F	2. F	3. T	4. T	5. T

6.6 The following are the features associated with the healing of open wounds:

1. The formation of granulation tissue
2. Infection
3. Migration of the surrounding epithelium
4. Giant cell formation
5. Contraction

10.5 The following conditions are particularly associated with the deposition of amyloid:

1. Gas gangrene
2. Leprosy
3. Osteomyelitis
4. Bronchiectasis
5. Pneumococcal pneumonia

7.35 The following infections are common in immunodeficient patients:

1. *Pneumocystis carinii*
2. Diphtheria
3. Poliomyelitis
4. Cytomegalovirus
5. *Candida albicans*

23.4 The compensatory mechanisms available to preserve the organism as a whole in the 'shock state' include:

1. autoregulation
2. a fall in the pO_2 of the blood
3. decreased pulmonary compliance
4. an increased sympathoadrenal discharge
5. haemoconcentration

17.35 Consecutive clot:

1. occurs in arteries distal to a thrombotic obstruction
2. occurs in the collateral branches of an artery following obstruction to the main vessel
3. occurs in veins after the cessation of blood flow
4. extends proximally to the entrance of the next venous tributary
5. is formed of coralline thrombus

23.3 The chief pathological and physiological changes in 'shock lung' include:

1. intra-alveolar oedema and extravasation of erythrocytes into the alveoli
2. increased pulmonary compliance
3. infection
4. alkalosis
5. patchy opacities on the plain X-ray of the chest

17.32 Thrombocytopenia:

1. may occur as an autoimmune phenomenon
2. is caused by sulphonamides
3. is associated with an increased bleeding time
4. is associated with an increased clotting time
5. the thromboplastin generation test is useful in its recognition

7.29 The following micro-organisms are obligate or facultative intracellular parasites:

1. *Mycobacterium tuberculosis*
2. *Clostridium welchii*
3. *Corynebacterium diphtheria*
4. *Leishmania tropica*
5. Herpes simplex

16.11 Acute heart failure occurs:

1. in rheumatic fever
2. in rheumatoid arthritis
3. in myxoedema
4. following myocardial infarction
5. in acute nephritis

2.9 The following are the chemical mediators involved in acute inflammation:

1. Complement
2. Histamine
3. Insulin
4. Bradykinin
5. Lymphokine

22.7 The following immunosuppressive agents are purine or pyrimidine analogues:

1. Cyclophosphamide
2. Azathioprine
3. Methotrexate
4. Actinomycin C
5. Prednisone

7.10 Antibodies may be detected *in vitro* by:

1. precipitation
2. complement fixation
3. lymphokine production
4. lymphocyte transformation test
5. radioimmunoassay

23.10 Serum levels of HBsAg may be high in:

1. lepromatous leprosy
2. tuberculosis
3. Down's syndrome
4. heroin addicts
5. malignant melanoma

3.2 The following belong to the mononuclear phagocyte system:

1. Macrophages
2. Mast cells
3. Epithelioid cells
4. Fibroblasts
5. Küpffer cells

7.26 The following are the chief characteristics of delayed hypersensitivity reactions:

1. The development of a polymorphonuclear leucocyte infiltrate
2. The reaction has reached its maximum intensity at 4 hours
3. An individual can be passively sensitised with serum
4. It is associated with increased T-lymphocyte function
5. Complement activation is an essential feature

7.22 The following are, or contain, autoantibodies:

1. Cryoglobulins
2. Rheumatoid factor
3. Migration inhibitory factor
4. Antinuclear factor
5. Transfer factor

20.10 Severe pyloric stenosis is accompanied by the following biochemical changes:

1. A fall in the effective blood volume
2. A fall in the concentration of plasma sodium
3. A rise in pCO_2
4. Hypotonic urine
5. Hyperkalaemia

17.25 The plasma prothrombin time is increased in:

1. hepatocellular disease
2. obstructive jaundice
3. haemophilia
4. Christmas disease
5. following splenectomy

10.6 Secondary amyloidosis occurs in the following conditions

1. Familial mediterranean fever
2. Thalassaemia
3. Sickle-cell disease
4. Multiple myeloma
5. Rheumatoid arthritis

14.10 The commonest tumours of the central nervous system arise from:

1. the meninges
2. primary tumours elsewhere in the body
3. neuroglia
4. the blood vessels
5. nerve cells.

Question number	Answer				
6.6	1. T	2. T	3. T	4. F	5. T
10.5	1. F	2. T	3. T	4. T	5. F
7.35	1. T	2. F	3. F	4. T	5. T
23.4	1. T	2. F	3. F	4. T	5. F
17.35	1. F	2. F	3. T	4. T	5. F
23.3	1. T	2. F	3. T	4. F	5. T
17.32	1. T	2. T	3. T	4. F	5. F
7.29	1. T	2. F	3. F	4. T	5. T
16.11	1. T	2. F	3. F	4. T	5. T
2.9	1. T	2. T	3. F	4. T	5. F
22.7	1. F	2. T	3. F	4. F	5. F
7.10	1. T	2. T	3. F	4. F	5. T
23.10	1. T	2. F	3. T	4. T	5. F
3.2	1. T	2. F	3. T	4. F	5. T
7.26	1. F	2. F	3. F	4. T	5. F
7.22	1. T	2. T	3. F	4. T	5. F
20.10	1. T	2. F	3. T	4. F	5. F
17.25	1. T	2. T	3. F	4. F	5. F
10.6	1. T	2. F	3. F	4. T	5. T
14.10	1. F	2. T	3. T	4. F	5. F

11.5 Haemosiderosis differs from haemochromatosis in that:

1. the former is more common in the Bantu
2. the latter is due to the excessive absorption of iron and the former to excessive dietary intake
3. in the former the excessive iron is mainly deposited in the parenchymal cells whereas in the latter the excess iron is deposited mainly in the macrophages of the liver, spleen and bone marrow
4. in the former cirrhosis does not develop
5. in the latter the level of plasma transferrin is abnormally high

3.9 Epithelioid cell granuloma formation is associated with the following diseases:

1. Ulcerative colitis
2. Crohn's disease
3. Chronic glomerulo-nephritis
4. Toxoplasmosis
5. Sarcoidosis

9.7 Osteoporosis differs from osteomalacia in that:

1. the radiographic density of the skeleton is reduced in the former and not the latter
2. the remaining bone in the former presents a normal histological appearance
3. major changes occur in the epiphyses in the former
4. pseudofractures are commoner in the former than the latter
5. excess osteoid tissue is present in the former

19.7 Uretero-colic anastomosis is followed by:

1. ascending pyelonephritis
2. absorption of ammonium salts
3. absorption of urea from the colon
4. metabolic alkalosis
5. hyperkalaemia

7.11 Hypogammaglobulinaemia may occur in the following conditions:

1. Prematurity
2. Gluten sensitivity enteropathy
3. Di George syndrome
4. Autoimmune thyroiditis
5. Hodgkin's lymphoma

20.2 The percentage of total body water in any individual is influenced by:

1. the lean body mass
2. the activity of the adrenal cortex
3. the sodium content of the diet
4. thyroid activity
5. vomiting

3.1 Necrosis occurs as a concomitant feature of chronic inflammation in:

1. leprosy
2. tuberculosis
3. syphilis
4. actinomycosis
5. coccidiomycosis

7.8 The germinal centres of lymph nodes:

1. participate in cell-mediated immunity
2. contain macrophages and plasma cells
3. originate in primary follicles
4. enlarge in chronic infectious diseases
5. are absent from the lymph nodes of mice subjected to thymectomy in the neonatal period and in children suffering from the Di George syndrome

20.5 Combined water and electrolyte depletion causes:

1. a high concentration of sodium in the urine
2. a high urine specific gravity
3. pre-renal uraemia
4. a fall in the central venous pressure
5. a high blood urea nitrogen to creatinine ratio

7.19 Serum sickness

1. can be caused by an injection of diphtheria anti-toxin
2. is caused by the injection of tetanus toxoid
3. is caused by the injection of penicillin
4. may be immune complex mediated
5. may be anaphylactic

6.5 Post operative infection delays wound healing because:

1. the wound becomes packed with leucocytes
2. many of the organisms involved produce spreading factors which may destroy the intercellular ground substance
3. collagen is destroyed
4. capillary loops fail to develop
5. fibroblasts are diminished in number

17.12 The following abnormalities occur in pernicious anaemia:

1. A low haemoglobin
2. A decreased mean corpuscular haemoglobin (MCH)
3. An increased reticulocyte count
4. Antibodies to the parietal cells of the stomach
5. A decrease in the circulating level of vitamin B_{12}

17.13 In pernicious anaemia the following pathological changes may be seen:

1. Haemosiderosis
2. Atrophy of the gastric mucosa
3. A decrease in the volume of red marrow in the long bones
4. Extramedullary haemopoiesis
5. Demyelination of the lateral and dorsal columns, not associated with gliosis

3.10 Organised epithelioid cell granulomas develop in the following infections:

1. Leprosy
2. Syphilis
3. Ankylostomiasis
4. Ascariasis
5. Schistosomiasis

15.1 The following are viral diseases:

1. Cytomegalic inclusion disease
2. Trachoma
3. Dengue
4. Primary atypical pneumonia
5. Typhus

12.1 Obstruction of the common bile duct is associated with the following biochemical abnormalities:

1. A greater increase in the serum concentration of bilirubin diglucuronide than bilirubin monoglucuronide
2. A decrease in the serum concentration of unconjugated bilirubin
3. A decrease in the faecal stercobilinogen content
4. An increase in faecal fat
5. An increase in urinary urobilinogen

17.28 Haemorrhagic lesions may occur as a result of:

1. vitamin B deficiency
2. vitamin C deficiency
3. retinol deficiency
4. the nephrotic syndrome
5. penicillin therapy

15.7 The following infections may be successfully prevented by the administration of a vaccine:

1. Herpes simplex
2. Rabies
3. Lassa fever
4. Poliomyelitis
5. Yellow fever

22.8 Chlorambucil, a potent cytotoxic agent, causes:

1. a cessation of DNA synthesis
2. indirect interference with mitosis
3. inhibition of purine synthesis
4. binding of DNA strands
5. inhibition of protein synthesis

18.8 The Zollinger Ellison syndrome is associated with:

1. β-cell tumours of the pancreas
2. chronic duodenal ulceration
3. cholereiform diarrhoea
4. parathyroid adenomata
5. phaeochromocytoma

Question number	Answer
11.5	1. T 2. F 3. F 4. T 5. F
3.9	1. F 2. T 3. F 4. T 5. T
9.7	1. F 2. T 3. F 4. F 5. F
19.7	1. T 2. T 3. T 4. F 5. F
7.11	1. T 2. T 3. F 4. F 5. T
20.2	1. T 2. T 3. F 4. T 5. T
3.1	1. F 2. T 3. T 4. T 5. T
7.8	1. F 2. T 3. T 4. T 5. F
20.5	1. F 2. T 3. T 4. T 5. F
7.19	1. T 2. F 3. T 4. T 5. T
6.5	1. F 2. F 3. T 4. F 5. F
17.12	1. T 2. F 3. F 4. T 5. T
17.13	1. T 2. T 3. F 4. T 5. T
3.10	1. T 2. T 3. F 4. F 5. T
15.1	1. T 2. F 3. T 4. F 5. F
12.1	1. F 2. F 3. T 4. T 5. F
17.28	1. F 2. T 3. F 4. F 5. T
15.7	1. F 2. T 3. F 4. T 5. T
22.8	1. F 2. T 3. F 4. T 5. T
18.8	1. F 2. T 3. T 4. T 5. F

7.18 The production of antibody is essential to host resistance in the following infection:

1. Leprosy
2. Pneumococcal pneumonia
3. Vaccinia
4. Tetanus
5. Malaria

13.10 The following substances are oncofoetal antigens:

1. HSA
2. α-fetoprotein
3. Bence Jones protein
4. Chorionic gonadotrophin
5. Carcinoembryonic antigen

2.14 Septicaemia is associated with:

1. a bacteraemia
2. toxaemia
3. the multiplication of bacteria in the blood stream
4. invasion of the blood stream by organisms multiplying elsewhere in the circulation, e.g. the peritoneum
5. multiple haemorrhagic foci in the tissues

2.10 The following substances are involved in acute inflammation:

1. Peptides
2. Lectins
3. Plasmin
4. LATS
5. PGE_1

17.20 Chronic lymphocytic leukaemia is associated with:

1. a marked increase in the number of lymphocytes in the peripheral blood
2. the early appearance of anaemia
3. an early bleeding tendency
4. an increase in the serum globulin concentration
5. an increase in the number of B-lymphocytes in the blood

4.2 General factors predisposing to wound infection include:

1. uncontrolled diabetes
2. hypogammaglobulinaemia
3. low platelet count
4. agranulocytopenia
5. eosinophilia

2.11 Phagocytosis is promoted by:

1. hyaluronidase
2. neuraminidase
3. the hexose monophosphate shunt
4. immunoglobulin
5. complement

17.31 Thrombocytopenia can be caused by:

1. deficiency of clotting factors
2. haemorrhage
3. diuretics
4. measles virus
5. telangiectasia

2.8 The main components of the pyogenic membrane are:

1. eosinophils
2. capillary loops
3. hyaluronidase
4. polymorphonuclear leucocytes
5. fibroblasts

6.7 Wound healing may be governed by the following:

1. Trephones
2. Vitamin D
3. Chalones
4. Mineralocorticoids
5. The availability of sulphur containing aminoacids

19.2 The renal control of acid base balance is a function of the:

1. loop of Henlé
2. proximal tubule
3. glomerulus
4. distal tubule
5. collecting tubule

2.1 Acute inflammation can be caused by:

1. *Streptococcus pneumoniae*
2. *Mycobacterium tuberculosis*
3. *Neisseria meningitidis*
4. *Mycobacterium leprae*
5. *Borrelia vincenti*

7.17 Complement activation takes place:

1. in the presence of endotoxin
2. as part of the tuberculin reaction
3. by more than one pathway
4. in anaphylaxis
5. by antigen IgA interaction

12.4 In liver failure the following biochemical abnormalities may be found:

1. A decrease in the plasma albumin concentration
2. An increase in the plasma globulin
3. An increase in the blood ammonium concentration
4. A rise in the blood urea
5. Impaired glucose tolerance

5.4 Chemical agents used as disinfectants and antiseptics include the following compounds:

1. The phenols
2. Isopropyl alcohol
3. The halogens
4. The soaps
5. Derivatives of salicylic acid

7.34 The following can cause immunological unresponsiveness:

1. Immunological tolerance
2. Immunological enhancement
3. Freund's adjuvant
4. T-lymphocytes
5. Antigen-antibody complexes

14.3 Neoplastic disease may be associated with the following conditions:

1. Dermatomyositis
2. Acanthosis nigricans
3. Necrobiosis lipoidica
4. Thrombophlebitis migrans
5. Polyarteritis nodosa

13.4 The following are carcinogenic:

1. Infra-red radiation
2. Ultra-violet radiation
3. House dust
4. Soot
5. Moulds

6.9 The healing of a closed fracture may be associated with the following pathological consequences:

1. Myositis ossificans
2. Pseudarthrosis
3. Osteomyelitis
4. Osteosarcoma
5. Renal calculi

16.3 The following conditions are associated with hyperlipidaemia:

1. Familial hypercholesteraemia
2. The nephrotic syndrome
3. Cushing's syndrome
4. Hyperaldosteronism
5. Thyrotoxicosis

Question number	Answer				
7.18	1. F	2. T	3. F	4. T	5. T
13.10	1. F	2. T	3. F	4. F	5. T
2.14	1. F	2. T	3. T	4. F	5. T
2.10	1. T	2. F	3. T	4. F	5. T
17.20	1. T	2. F	3. F	4. F	5. T
4.2	1. T	2. T	3. T	4. T	5. F
2.11	1. F	2. F	3. F	4. T	5. T
17.31	1. F	2. T	3. T	4. T	5. F
2.8	1. F	2. T	3. F	4. T	5. T
6.7	1. T	2. F	3. T	4. F	5. T
19.2	1. F	2. F	3. F	4. T	5. F
2.1	1. T	2. T	3. T	4. F	5. T
7.17	1. T	2. F	3. T	4. F	5. F
12.4	1. T	2. T	3. T	4. F	5. T
5.4	1. T	2. T	3. T	4. T	5. F
7.34	1. T	2. T	3. F	4. F	5. T
14.3	1. T	2. T	3. F	4. T	5. F
13.4	1. F	2. T	3. F	4. T	5. T
6.9	1. T	2. T	3. F	4. F	5. T
16.3	1. T	2. T	3. T	4. F	5. F

7.9 Lymphokines, soluble factors released from primed lymphocytes in contact with an antigen are important in:

1. anaphylaxis
2. immune complex disease
3. macrophage activation
4. macrophage migratory inhibition
5. lymphocyte mitogenesis

12.9 Severe liver failure is associated with:

1. mucosal bleeding
2. encephalopathy
3. bronchopneumonia
4. venous thrombosis
5. decreased resistance to infection

18.3 An eosinophil adenoma of the anterior hypophysis is associated with:

1. enlargement of the sella turcica
2. hypertrophy and hyperplasia of the soft tissues throughout the body
3. excessive growth of the acral parts
4. premature closure of the epiphyses
5. impaired glucose tolerance

15.6 The Hepatitis B virus:

1. is transmitted by the oral route
2. is transmitted by dogs
3. is common in renal dialysis units
4. is the cause of Burkitt's lymphoma
5. causes immune complex disease

21.7 The Coombs test is used for detecting:

1. rheumatoid factor
2. antinuclear factor
3. haemolytic autoantibodies
4. cold agglutinins
5. rhesus antibodies

15.2 Encephalitis may be a complication of the following virus infections:

1. Epstein Barr virus
2. Measles virus
3. Rubella virus
4. Herpes virus
5. Adenovirus

17.29 Disseminated intravascular coagulation is a complication of:

1. surgical operations such as prostatectomy or open heart surgery
2. malignant disease
3. thrombocythaemia
4. the overadministration of thrombokinase
5. endotoxaemic shock

9.3 The destruction of bone is associated with the following biochemical changes:

1. An increased secretion of hydroxyproline in the urine
2. An elevated alkaline phosphatase
3. An elevated acid phosphatase
4. An elevated serum calcium
5. Depression of the serum phosphate

7.7 Autoimmunity

1. occurs because of a breakdown in the ability of the body to distinguish between self and non-self
2. is involved in some forms of orchitis
3. is involved in the production of cryoglobulins
4. is important in the pathogenesis of lupus erythematosus
5. does not result in immune complex disease

14.7 The findings of the following substances in excessive quantities in the blood may be due to the presence of a specific type of tumour:

1. Noradrenaline
2. 5-hydroxytryptamine
3. Carcinoembryonic antigen
4. Prostaglandins
5. Calcium

17.19 Chronic myeloid leukaemia differs from chronic lymphatic leukaemia in that:

1. in the former the predominant white cell in the circulation is the leucocyte
2. the total white count is higher in chronic lymphatic leukaemia
3. in the former the proliferating marrow cells possess the Philadelphia chromosome
4. the latter is more common in an older age group than is the former
5. the former disease tends to develop into a more aggressive type of acute leukaemia

2.7 The magnitude of leucocyte migration into an area infected with bacteria is governed by:

1. the type of organism causing the inflammatory lesion
2. chemotaxins
3. the C5a complement component
4. the phosphatase levels in the inflamed area
5. the formation of pus

10.8 Amyloidosis may be associated with elevated levels of the following serum proteins:

1. β-lipoprotein
2. SAA
3. IgD
4. M-protein
5. β-microglobulin

18.5 Abnormal aggregation of lymphocytes occurs in the thyroid in the following pathological conditions:

1. Follicular carcinoma
2. Medullary carcinoma
3. Lymphadenoid goitre
4. Reidel's struma
5. Primary thyrotoxicosis

23.9 Chromosome abnormalities may occur:

1. in Klinefelter's syndrome
2. following treatment with methotrexate
3. as a result of ionising radiation
4. in Down's syndrome
5. in Christmas disease

2.4 The blood flow through acutely inflamed tissues is decreased by the following events:

1. Increased cellular concentration in the blood flowing through the inflamed part
2. Loss of protein from the dilated capillaries
3. Aggregation of the red cells
4. Adherence of leucocytes to the capillary endothelium
5. Lewis' axon reflex

7.27 Maximum changes occur in the following skin reactions within 24 to 48 hours:

1. Schwartzmann reaction
2. Arthus reaction
3. Tuberculin reaction
4. Contact patch test
5. Skin allograft rejection

14.6 Exfoliative cytology is useful for the diagnosis of:

1. meningioma
2. bronchial cancer
3. multiple myeloma
4. cervical cancer
5. vesical cancer

23.1 The following are referred to as 'Incomplete Antibodies':

1. IgG anti-D
2. IgM anti-D
3. Anti-A isohaemagglutinin
4. The Wassermann antibody
5. Tetanus antitoxin

14.5 The following tumours may secrete hormones:

1. Carcinoid tumours
2. Choriocarcinoma
3. Arrhenoblastoma
4. Teratoma
5. Seminoma

Question number	Answer
7.9	1. F 2. F 3. T 4. T 5. T
12.9	1. T 2. T 3. T 4. F 5. T
18.3	1. T 2. T 3. T 4. F 5. T
15.6	1. T 2. F 3. T 4. F 5. T
21.7	1. F 2. F 3. T 4. T 5. T
15.2	1. T 2. T 3. T 4. T 5. F
17.29	1. T 2. T 3. T 4. F 5. T
9.3	1. T 2. T 3. F 4. T 5. T
7.7	1. T 2. T 3. T 4. T 5. F
14.7	1. T 2. T 3. T 4. F 5. T
17.19	1. T 2. F 3. T 4. F 5. T
2.7	1. T 2. T 3. T 4. F 5. T
10.8	1. F 2. T 3. F 4. T 5. F
18.5	1. F 2. F 3. T 4. F 5. T
23.9	1. T 2. F 3. T 4. T 5. F
2.4	1. T 2. F 3. T 4. T 5. F
7.27	1. F 2. F 3. T 4. T 5. F
14.6	1. F 2. T 3. F 4. T 5. T
23.1	1. T 2. F 3. F 4. F 5. F
14.5	1. F 2. T 3. T 4. T 5. F

3.8 Direct evidence of immunological activity can be demonstrated in the following chronic inflammatory diseases:

1. Lepromatous leprosy
2. Tuberculoid leprosy
3. Silicosis
4. Rheumatoid arthritis
5. Asbestosis

2.13 Pus contains:

1. lipids
2. fibrin
3. collagen
4. plasma cells
5. polymorphonuclear leucocytes

5.3 Differences between disinfectants and antiseptics are as follows:

1. The latter are more harmful to living tissue cells
2. Antiseptics free inanimate objects from vegetative organisms whereas disinfectants are used for the local removal of pathogenic bacteria from the tissues
3. The former are more readily inactivated by contact with proteinaceous material such as blood
4. The speed of action of the former can be accelerated by raising the temperature whereas the action of the latter can only be increased by increasing their concentration
5. There are specific differences in the mode of action of both groups of compounds

4.8 The major pathogens in post operative chest infections are:

1. *Haemophilus influenzae*
2. *Streptococcus pyogenes*
3. *Mycobacterium tuberculosis*
4. *Staphylococcus aureus*
5. *Streptococcus pneumoniae*

22.5 The following compounds may be used as anti-cancer agents:

1. Azathioprine
2. Methotrexate
3. Actinomycin D
4. Chlorambucil
5. Cyclosporin A

21.4 An immediate reaction to a blood transfusion may be caused by the following:

1. Hypercalcaemia
2. Air embolus
3. Bacterial endotoxins
4. Anaphylaxis
5. Hypokalaemia

14.12 The interphase is:

1. situated between the prophase and metaphase
2. a resting stage between cell division
3. associated with growth of a cell
4. accompanied by the accumulation of RNA
5. situated between the anaphase and the telophase

3.7 The following predispose to the development of tuberculosis:

1. HLA – B27
2. Sarcoidosis
3. Silicosis
4. Avitaminosis D
5. Malnutrition

16.10 The following congenital anomalies of the heart are accompanied by continuous cyanosis:

1. Complete transposition of the great vessels
2. Uncomplicated patent ductus arteriosus
3. Coarctation of the aorta
4. Double aortic arch
5. Tetralogy of Fallot

19.4 The nephrotic syndrome is accompanied by:

1. decreased glomerular capillary permeability
2. oedema
3. a loss of 10 g or more of plasma protein daily
4. hypolipidaemia
5. abundant cortical deposits of neutral fat and anisotropic lipids

3.6 Giant cells are characteristically found in the pathological lesions associated with the following diseases:

1. Actinomycosis
2. Schistosomiasis
3. Primary biliary cirrhosis
4. Lepromatous leprosy
5. Hodgkin's disease

4.6 Bacteria are normally found on or in the:

1. blood
2. urinary tract
3. lower bronchi
4. gastrointestinal tract
5. skin, sebaceous glands and hair follicles

2.2 The following agents produce an acute inflammatory reaction in unsensitised individuals:

1. Lipopolysaccharide
2. Albumin
3. Ultra-violet light
4. Insulin
5. Carbon particles

9.4 Hypercalcaemia and hypercalciuria is caused by:

1. osteolytic secondary deposits in bone
2. hypervitaminosis D, often referred to as vitamin D intoxication
3. parathyroid tumours
4. tumours of adrenal medulla
5. primary carcinoma of the kidney restricted to the kidney

16.2 Cholesterol is believed to be of great importance in the development of atherosclerosis because:

1. low plasma cholesterol concentrations are associated with relative freedom from atherosclerotic heart disease
2. high concentrations of cholesterol occur in the atherosclerotic plaques
3. patients suffering from steatorrhoea develop atherosclerosis at a younger age than normal individuals
4. diabetes is associated with an increased incidence of atherosclerosis
5. atherosclerosis can be induced in non-human primates by dietary measures which increase the concentration of cholesterol in the plasma

5.9 Ototoxicity is a well recognised complication following the administration of:

1. Streptomycin
2. Gentamicin
3. Neomycin
4. Bacitracin
5. Erythromycin

13.7 The following infections are associated with the development of cancer:

1. Clostridial infections
2. HBV infection
3. EBV infection
4. Chlamydial infections
5. Schistosomiasis

22.2 The effect(s) of ionising irradiation:

1. are increased by sulphydryl reagents
2. are increased by increased oxygen tension
3. is mainly upon mitochondria
4. is to cause diarrhoea
5. is to cause a deficiency of clotting factors

17.34 Thrombocytopenic purpura differs from non-thrombocytopenic purpura in that:

1. in the former condition the platelet count is reduced
2. in the latter the main defect is in the capillaries
3. the former may follow systemic disease
4. the latter may result from allergy
5. petechiae occur in the former but not in the latter

7.15 The third component of complement is:

1. a factor in phagocytosis
2. an anaphylatoxin
3. chemotactic
4. migration inhibition factor
5. an interferon

Question number	Answer				
3.8	1. F	2. T	3. F	4. T	5. F
2.13	1. T	2. T	3. F	4. F	5. T
5.3	1. F	2. F	3. F	4. F	5. F
4.8	1. T	2. F	3. F	4. T	5. T
22.5	1. F	2. T	3. T	4. T	5. F
21.4	1. F	2. T	3. T	4. T	5. F
14.12	1. F	2. T	3. T	4. T	5. F
3.7	1. F	2. F	3. F	4. F	5. T
16.10	1. T	2. F	3. F	4. F	5. T
19.4	1. F	2. T	3. T	4. F	5. T
3.6	1. F	2. F	3. T	4. F	5. T
4.6	1. F	2. F	3. F	4. T	5. T
2.2	1. T	2. F	3. T	4. F	5. F
9.4	1. T	2. T	3. T	4. F	5. F
16.2	1. T	2. T	3. F	4. F	5. T
5.9	1. T	2. T	3. T	4. F	5. F
13.7	1. F	2. T	3. T	4. F	5. T
22.2	1. F	2. T	3. F	4. T	5. F
17.34	1. T	2. T	3. T	4. T	5. F
7.15	1. T	2. T	3. T	4. F	5. F

20.1 The major differences between the plasma and the interstitial fluid are in:

1. the concentration of sodium
2. the concentration of calcium
3. the bicarbonate concentration
4. the protein content
5. the organic acid concentration

13.1 A hereditary predisposition to the development of tumours occurs at the following sites:

1. Retina
2. Colon
3. Lung
4. Skin
5. Stomach

14.1 A tumour may be defined as:

1. An abnormal mass of tissue
2. A growth of tissue which exceeds and is unco-ordinated with that of normal tissues
3. A growth of tissue which is limited and co-ordinated with that of the rest of the body
4. An abnormal increase in the cells of a tissue
5. A malformation in which the various tissues of the part are present in improper proportions or distribution

15.3 Inclusion bodies are found in the following viral infections:

1. Zoster
2. Yellow fever
3. Rabies
4. Hepatitis B
5. Smallpox

17.10 Polycythaemia occurs in:

1. congenital cyanotic heart disease
2. tumours of the renal parenchyma, renal carcinoma
3. the carcinoid syndrome
4. lead poisoning
5. hypoxia

9.5 Excessive osteoid tissue is formed in:

1. vitamin D deficiency
2. Muslim women
3. patients on anticonvulsant drugs
4. patients on long term anticoagulant therapy
5. long-standing obstructive jaundice

14.13 The embryonic tumours of infancy include:

1. nephroblastoma
2. osteogenic sarcoma (osteosarcoma)
3. medulloblastoma
4. cholangiocarcinoma
5. lympho-epithelioma

23.5 Which among the following are protozoal infections:

1. Hydatid disease
2. Trypanosomiasis
3. Giardiasis
4. Schistosomiasis
5. Filariasis

3.4 Accumulation of macrophages is a prominent histological feature of the lesions produced by the following diseases:

1. Leishmaniasis
2. Extrinsic allergic alveolitis
3. Gaucher's disease
4. Legionnaire's disease
5. Letterer-Siwe's disease

10.9 Amyloid reacts with the following stains:

1. Thioflavine-T
2. Fluoroscein isothiocyanate
3. Methyl violet
4. Methyl green
5. Congo red

17.22 An enlarged lymph node which is excised is found by histological examination to be packed with tubercles consisting of epithelioid cells and giant cells. The tuberculin and Heaf test are negative. Which of the following diseases should then be considered as the probable cause of the lymphadenopathy?

1. Hodgkin's disease
2. Tuberculosis
3. Sarcoidosis
4. Syphilis
5. Toxoplasmosis

9.8 Urinary hydroxyproline excretion may be increased in:

1. Paget's disease of bone
2. Cushing's syndrome
3. hypopituitarism in children
4. hyperthyroidism
5. extensive fractures

17.11 Megaloblastic anaemia may be caused by:

1. atrophy or ablation of the gastric mucosa
2. infestation with *Diphyllobothrium latum*
3. lesions involving the terminal ileum
4. over-enthusiastic use of purgatives
5. small bowel blind loops

5.7 Bacteria resistant to benzyl penicillin include:

1. penicillinase-producing organisms
2. the majority of Gram-negative bacteria
3. Gram-positive anaerobic spore forming organisms
4. the Bacteroides
5. *Streptococcus pneumoniae*

20.6 Pure water depletion in the surgical patient follows:

1. persistent vomiting
2. dysphagia
3. severe diarrhoea
4. persistent fever
5. the development of diabetes insipidus

9.6 The sites in which metastatic calcification occurs are:

1. the pyramids of the kidney
2. the wall of the inferior vena cava
3. old tuberculous lesions
4. atheroma
5. the cornea

7.31 The following cells play an important role in skin allograft rejection:

1. Polymorphonuclear leucocytes
2. Macrophages
3. Mast cells
4. B-lymphocytes
5. T-lymphocytes

2.6 The following cell types are involved in acute inflammation:

1. Polymorphonuclear leucocytes
2. Lymphocytes
3. Endothelial cells
4. Epithelioid cells
5. Mast cells

1.1 Disuse atrophy follows:

1. blockage of the duct of an exocrine gland
2. immobilisation of a joint
3. interference with the nerve supply to the muscles controlling joint movement
4. interference with the blood supply
5. the diminished secretion of trophic hormones

17.2 Alterations in the structure of the Hb molecule give rise to the following diseases:

1. Haemolytic disease of the newborn
2. Sickle-cell anaemia
3. Paroxysmal cold haemoglobinuria
4. Paroxysmal nocturnal haemoglobinuria
5. Thalassaemia major

Question number			Answer		
20.1	1. T	2. F	3. F	4. T	5. F
13.1	1. T	2. T	3. F	4. T	5. F
14.1	1. T	2. T	3. F	4. F	5. F
15.3	1. T	2. F	3. T	4. F	5. T
17.10	1. T	2. T	3. F	4. F	5. T
9.5	1. T	2. T	3. T	4. F	5. T
14.13	1. T	2. F	3. T	4. F	5. F
23.5	1. F	2. T	3. F	4. F	5. F
3.4	1. T	2. F	3. T	4. F	5. T
10.9	1. T	2. F	3. T	4. F	5. T
17.22	1. F	2. F	3. T	4. F	5. F
9.8	1. T	2. F	3. F	4. T	5. T
17.11	1. T	2. T	3. T	4. F	5. T
5.7	1. T	2. F	3. F	4. T	5. F
20.6	1. F	2. T	3. F	4. T	5. T
9.6	1. T	2. F	3. F	4. F	5. T
7.31	1. F	2. T	3. F	4. F	5. T
2.6	1. T	2. F	3. T	4. F	5. T
1.1	1. T	2. T	3. F	4. F	5. F
17.2	1. F	2. T	3. F	4. F	5. T

7.6 Macrophages:

1. are not involved in the recognition of antigens
2. do not secrete lysosomal enzymes
3. can carry antibody on their surface
4. are involved in the tuberculin reaction
5. are important in graft rejection

11.2 Patchy skin pigmentation occurs in the following conditions:

1. Peutz–Jegher syndrome
2. Familial polyposis
3. Addison's disease
4. Purpura
5. Vitiligo

9.9 The following pathological changes can occur in metabolic bone disease:

1. Osteoporosis
2. Localized areas of skeletal involvement
3. Osteomalacia
4. Osteopetrosis
5. Osteitis fibrosa cystica

23.6 Mosquitoes transmit the following diseases:

1. Schistosomiasis
2. Leishmaniasis
3. Dengue
4. Yellow Fever
5. Malaria

18.10 Diabetes insipidus is associated with:

1. the oversecretion of vasopressin
2. polydipsia
3. a urine specific gravity greater than 1020
4. head injury
5. metastatic cancer

4.9 The following bacteria are commonly found in infected wounds following colonic operations:

1. *Escherichia coli*
2. *Neisseriae meningitidis*
3. *Streptococcus pyogenes*
4. *Streptococcus faecalis*
5. *Bacteroides fragilis*

20.3 The renin-angiotensin-aldosterone system regulates:

1. potassium balance
2. sodium balance
3. fluid volume
4. blood pressure
5. nitrogen balance

9.1 The normal level of ionised calcium in the plasma is maintained by the following mechanisms:

1. The secretion of calcitonin
2. The presence of 1,25 $(OH)_2$ D_3
3. Parathyroid hormone secretion
4. Renal tubular conservation
5. The circulating level of magnesium

7.13 The Arthus reaction:

1. is associated with marked emigration of polymorphonuclear leucocytes into the surrounding tissues
2. is not associated with complement activation
3. is a delayed hypersensitivity reaction
4. is associated with vascular damage
5. is produced by endotoxin

11.1 Generalised pigmentation of the skin occurs in:

1. carcinoma of the head of the pancreas
2. idiopathic haemochromatosis
3. argyria
4. arsenic poisoning
5. black liver disease

14.9 Hormone dependency may be exhibited by the following tumours:

1. Malignant melanoma
2. Prostatic carcinoma
3. Follicular carcinoma of the thyroid
4. Bronchial carcinoma
5. Retinoblastoma

12.7 The main constituents of gall stones are:

1. calcium sulphate
2. cholesterol
3. calcium palmitate
4. calcium bilirubinate
5. amorphous materials

22.6 The following compounds are alkylating agents:

1. Azathioprine
2. Methotrexate
3. Cyclophosphamide
4. Phenylalanine mustard
5. Tetracycline

7.4 T-lymphocytes:

1. are immunoglobulin-secreting cells
2. are found in the paracortical area of lymph nodes
3. are involved in contact dermatitis
4. are not involved in protection against tuberculosis
5. secrete lymphokines

15.4 The following are RNA containing viruses:

1. Rhinovirus
2. Herpes virus
3. Vaccinia
4. Yellow Fever
5. Influenza

13.6 The following occupations have been, or remain associated with, a high incidence of cancer:

1. Coal mining
2. Nickel workers
3. Asbestos workers
4. Dye industry
5. Tobacco industry

20.9 Hypocalcaemia occurs:

1. following surgical damage or removal of the parathyroid glands
2. following fractures of the long bones
3. during attacks of acute pancreatitis
4. following head injury
5. in association with hypomagnesaemia

7.2 The following statements are true or false:

1. IgA is produced at mucous surfaces
2. IgM has a molecular weight 150 000
3. IgE is the anaphylactic antibody
4. Antibody specificity depends on the constant regions of the F(ab) fragment
5. Immunoglobulin synthesis is dependent on thymic integrity in neonatal life

7.38 Haptoglobins:

1. bind to the body's own proteins to make them immunogenic
2. are immunoglobulins
3. bind to free haemoglobin
4. are controlled by genetic factors
5. can bind rheumatoid factor

13.5 The following chemicals are carcinogens:

1. 3.4 benzpyrene
2. 2.4 dinitrofluorobenzene
3. β-naphthylamine
4. Acetyl salicyclic acid
5. 4-dimethylamino-azobenzene

Question number		Answer			
7.6	1. F	2. F	3. T	4. T	5. T
11.2	1. T	2. F	3. F	4. T	5. F
9.9	1. T	2. F	3. T	4. T	5. T
23.6	1. F	2. F	3. T	4. T	5. T
18.10	1. F	2. T	3. F	4. T	5. T
4.9	1. T	2. F	3. T	4. T	5. T
20.3	1. T	2. T	3. T	4. T	5. F
9.1	1. T	2. T	3. T	4. T	5. F
7.13	1. T	2. F	3. F	4. T	5. F
11.1	1. T	2. T	3. T	4. F	5. F
14.9	1. T	2. T	3. T	4. F	5. F
12.7	1. F	2. T	3. T	4. T	5. T
22.6	1. F	2. F	3. T	4. T	5. F
7.4	1. F	2. T	3. T	4. F	5. T
15.4	1. T	2. F	3. F	4. T	5. T
13.6	1. F	2. T	3. T	4. T	5. F
20.9	1. T	2. T	3. T	4. F	5. T
7.2	1. T	2. F	3. T	4. F	5. F
7.38	1. F	2. F	3. T	4. T	5. F
13.5	1. T	2. F	3. T	4. F	5. T

20.4 The blood urea is elevated in the following conditions:

1. Severe dehydration
2. Pregnancy
3. Tubular necrosis
4. Diabetes insipidus
5. Cortical necrosis

7.5 The major histocompatibility complex (MHC) in man:

1. is situated in chromosome 6
2. has three loci controlling five groups of histocompatibility antigens
3. is involved in the expression of immune response (Ir) genes
4. shows a positive association with Hodgkin's disease, multiple sclerosis and ankylosing spondylitis
5. is tested for by the laboratory on a serum sample

7.37 A non-specific depression of the tuberculin reaction occurs in:

1. influenza
2. measles
3. sarcoidosis
4. leprosy
5. ulcerative colitis

13.2 Recognised precancerous conditions include:

1. the intestinal polyps of the small bowel occurring in the Peutz–Jegher syndrome
2. the colonic polyps of familial polyposis
3. Xeroderma pigmentosum
4. Bowen's disease
5. Molluscum sebaceum

12.6 Excessive cholesterol is excreted by the hepatocytes:

1. when the diet contains excessive amounts of polyunsaturated fatty acids
2. in response to excessive secretion of testosterone
3. when an individual is excessively obese
4. when anticoagulants are administered in large doses
5. when calorie intake is diminished

7.23 Antiglobulins are involved in the:

1. Wassermann reaction
2. Coombs test
3. fluorescent antibody test
4. rheumatoid factor test
5. Casoni test

18.1 Phaeochromocytoma may be associated with:

1. paroxysmal hypertension
2. sweating
3. neurofibromatosis
4. a fall in blood pressure on palpating the abdomen
5. paroxysmal hypotension

12.3 The common causes of cirrhosis of the liver in Great Britain are:

1. alcohol
2. various drugs such as halothane and paracetamol
3. active chronic hepatitis
4. haemochromatosis
5. cryptogenic

3.3 Malignant disease may complicate the following chronic inflammatory diseases:

1. Chronic osteomyelitis
2. Sarcoidosis
3. Asbestosis
4. Schistosomiasis
5. Ulcerative colitis

7.36 The following conditions are associated with T-cell immunodeficiency:

1. Hodgkin's disease
2. Tay-Sachs disease
3. Wiskott Aldrich syndrome
4. Down's syndrome
5. Di George syndrome

16.12 Left sided heart failure occurs as a complication of:

1. hypertension
2. mitral regurgitation
3. pulmonary fibrosis
4. uncomplicated coronary atherosclerosis
5. tricuspid stenosis

6.10 Ischaemic necrosis is a recognised complication of fractures of the following bones:

1. Talus
2. Calcaneum
3. Scaphoid
4. Pisiform
5. Femoral head

19.6 The differences between the tubular lesions produced by nephrotoxic drugs and renal ischaemia include the following:

1. The lesion produced by ischaemia occurs in a random fashion throughout all nephrons and in any part of the nephron down to collecting tubules
2. A nephrotoxic drug affects the entire nephron
3. Nephrotoxic drugs produce scattered lesions throughout the kidney
4. Ischaemia causes complete necrosis of the tubule cell together with the basement membrane
5. Nephrotoxins cause both cytotoxic and ischaemic lesions

15.5 The Epstein Barr virus is associated with:

1. glandular fever
2. the Australia antigen
3. Burkitt's lymphoma
4. nasopharyngeal carcinoma
5. the common cold

6.4 Collagen, the ultimate source of the strength of a wound:

1. is formed by undifferentiated mesenchymal cells
2. is changed with the passage of time
3. undergoes lysis as well as synthesis even when the total collagen content of the wound is remaining constant
4. is broken down by the enzyme collagenase
5. is normally embedded in ground substance

4.10 The incidence of postoperative infection can be reduced by the use of the following measures:

1. The use of negative pressure ventilation in the operating theatre
2. The use of filtered air in the operating theatre, pore size 10 μm
3. Showering by the surgeon and all attendants prior to embarking upon the operation
4. The administration of prophylactic antibiotics
5. Disinfection of the patient's skin prior to operation

7.21 An autoimmune haemolytic anaemia:

1. does not occur in systemic lupus erythematosus
2. does not show Rhesus specificity
3. may be associated with mycoplasma infection
4. may be caused by drug therapy
5. is not associated with leucopenia

22.3 Ionising radiation:

1. does not affect the eyes
2. affects renal function
3. does not affect the lungs
4. affects the brain
5. does not affect the skin

1.6 Metaplasia, the transformation of one fully differentiated tissue into another, occurs in:

1. connective tissue elements
2. the gastrointestinal tract
3. the central nervous system
4. the biliary system
5. the urothelium

7.12 Active immunity can be produced by an appropriate vaccine to the following diseases:

1. Pneumococcal pneumonia
2. Plague
3. Chicken pox
4. Poliomyelitis
5. Typhoid

Question number			Answer		
20.4	1. T	2. F	3. T	4. F	5. T
7.5	1. T	2. F	3. T	4. T	5. F
7.37	1. F	2. T	3. T	4. T	5. F
13.2	1. F	2. T	3. T	4. T	5. F
12.6	1. T	2. F	3. T	4. F	5. F
7.23	1. F	2. T	3. T	4. T	5. F
18.1	1. T	2. T	3. T	4. F	5. T
12.3	1. T	2. F	3. T	4. F	5. T
3.3	1. T	2. F	3. T	4. T	5. T
7.36	1. T	2. F	3. T	4. F	5. T
16.12	1. T	2. T	3. F	4. T	5. F
6.10	1. T	2. F	3. T	4. F	5. T
19.6	1. T	2. F	3. F	4. T	5. T
15.5	1. T	2. F	3. T	4. T	5. F
6.4	1. F	2. T	3. T	4. T	5. T
4.10	1. F	2. F	3. F	4. T	5. T
7.21	1. F	2. F	3. T	4. T	5. F
22.3	1. F	2. T	3. F	4. T	5. F
1.6	1. T	2. T	3. F	4. T	5. T
7.12	1. F	2. T	3. F	4. T	5. T

6.3 The healing of a wound is delayed by:

1. vitamin C deficiency
2. starvation
3. the administration of glucocorticoids
4. lack of blood supply
5. infection

7.32 The following substances are lymphokines:

1. Properdin
2. Migration inhibitory factor
3. Macrophage chemotactic factor
4. Factor B
5. Interferon

16.8 Acquired syphilis of the cardiovascular system may involve the following lesions:

1. Myocardial gummata
2. Aortitis
3. Aortic regurgitation
4. Abdominal aortic aneurysm
5. Stenosis of the coronary ostia

5.2 Spores are killed by exposure to:

1. moist heat at 110°C for 15 minutes
2. dry heat at 160°C for 1 hour
3. ethylene oxide
4. hydrogen peroxide
5. gentian violet

15.8 The following viral infections are controlled by cell-mediated immunity:

1. Herpes simplex
2. Cytomegalic inclusion disease
3. Poliomyelitis
4. ECHO virus
5. Vaccinia

18.9 The following tumours of the ovary secrete hormones:

1. Arrhenoblastoma
2. Dysgerminoma
3. Dermoid cysts
4. Papillary cystadenoma
5. Granulosa-theca cell tumour

19.3 In renal tubular acidosis the following biochemical abnormalities occur:

1. An inability to lower the urine pH
2. Abnormal ammonia excretion in relation to urine pH
3. Renal glycosuria
4. Hypercalciuria
5. Hyperkalaemia

17.33 Platelets contribute to haemostasis by liberating:

1. 5-hydroxytryptamine (serotonin)
2. phospholipids
3. plasminogen
4. bradykinin
5. calcitonin

5.5 The following antibiotics are effective against fungi:

1. Nystatin
2. Bacitracin
3. Griseofulvin
4. Polymyxin B
5. Amphotericin B

7.28 Cell-mediated immune processes are of great importance in the control of the following infections:

1. Pneumococcal pneumonia
2. Diphtheria
3. Tuberculosis
4. Candidiasis
5. Mumps

19.8 Haemoglobinuria occurs:

1. in blackwater fever
2. following the excessive ingestion of beetroot
3. in any cause of haematuria when the specific gravity of the urine is above 1007
4. in blood transfusion
5. in strenuous exercise

21.6 Haemolytic disease of the newborn:

1. may be caused by *Treponema pallidum*
2. may be due to anti-c
3. may occur in the first pregnancy
4. frequently is not found until the second pregnancy
5. is treated with anti-D antibodies

22.1 Ionising radiation:

1. increases DNA synthesis
2. increases H_2O_2 in the tissues
3. breaks disulphide bonds
4. causes atrophy of the seminiferous tubules of the testis
5. causes pathological fractures

18.6 Primary hyperparathyroidism is associated with:

1. bone cysts
2. carcinoma of the parathyroid glands
3. dystrophic calcification
4. hypertension
5. anorexia

8.5 The following conditions are associated with a polyclonal gammopathy:

1. Waldenström's macroglobulinaemia
2. Rheumatoid arthritis
3. Down's syndrome
4. Wiskott Aldrich syndrome
5. Cirrhosis of the liver

10.2 Angioneurotic oedema, which is a neurovascular event, is associated with:

1. depression
2. complement deficiency
3. immunoglobulin E
4. menstruation
5. Lawrence's transfer factor

14.4 General phenomena associated with neoplasia may include:

1. fever
2. cachexia
3. thrombotic episodes
4. polycythaemia
5. dermatomyositis

19.5 The causes of acute tubular necrosis of the kidney include:

1. severe dehydration
2. the overadministration of carbon tetrachloride
3. acute porphyria
4. the overadministration of potassium chloride
5. gentamicin

17.6 Pathological destruction of red blood cells can take place in the following sites:

1. The submucosal plexus of the small intestine
2. The peripheral circulation
3. The liver
4. The spleen
5. The bone marrow

1.5 Starvation is associated with a reduction in size of the:

1. fat depots
2. heart
3. central nervous system
4. liver
5. bones

Question number			Answer		
6.3	1. T	2. T	3. T	4. T	5. T
7.32	1. F	2. T	3. T	4. F	5. T
16.8	1. T	2. T	3. T	4. F	5. T
5.2	1. F	2. T	3. T	4. F	5. F
15.8	1. T	2. T	3. F	4. F	5. T
18.9	1. T	2. T	3. T	4. F	5. T
19.3	1. T	2. F	3. F	4. T	5. F
17.33	1. T	2. T	3. F	4. F	5. F
5.5	1. T	2. F	3. T	4. F	5. T
7.28	1. F	2. F	3. T	4. T	5. T
19.8	1. T	2. F	3. F	4. F	5. T
21.6	1. F	2. T	3. T	4. T	5. T
22.1	1. F	2. T	3. F	4. T	5. T
18.6	1. T	2. T	3. F	4. T	5. T
8.5	1. F	2. T	3. F	4. F	5. T
10.2	1. F	2. T	3. T	4. F	5. F
14.4	1. T	2. T	3. T	4. T	5. T
19.5	1. T	2. T	3. T	4. F	5. F
17.6	1. F	2. T	3. T	4. T	5. T
1.5	1. T	2. T	3. F	4. T	5. F

19.1 Renal function is depressed in the following conditions:

1. 'Shock'
2. Amyloidosis
3. Chronic hyperuricaemia
4. Irradiation
5. Hypercalcaemia

14.8 Neuroblastoma are most common in:

1. children
2. adults
3. the adrenal medulla
4. the floor of the fourth ventricle
5. sympathetic ganglia

7.20 Anaphylactic reactions commonly follow the administration of the following drugs:

1. Penicillin
2. Azathioprine
3. Procaine
4. Alpha methyl-dopa
5. Hydralazine

23.8 Autosomal dominant diseases which are important to surgeons include:

1. hereditary spherocytosis
2. haemophilia
3. Von Recklinghausen's disease
4. familial agammaglobulinaemia
5. mucoviscidosis

8.2 The nephrotic syndrome is associated with:

1. no evidence of sodium retention
2. high levels of aldosterone in the urine
3. high levels of antidiuretic hormone in the urine
4. an increased blood volume
5. hypolipidaemia

2.5 The magnitude of the exudate associated with acute inflammation depends upon:

1. changes in the endothelium of the capillaries and venules
2. lymphocyte activation
3. the osmotic pressure of the plasma proteins
4. the plasma Ca^{++} level
5. the plasma K^+ level

13.8 An increase in the frequency of malignant disease occurs in the following conditions:

1. Following the long term administration of immunosuppressive agents
2. Large bowel Crohn's disease
3. Coeliac disease
4. Ulcerative colitis
5. Xeroderma pigmentosum

2.3 Normally the features of acute inflammation include:

1. vasoconstriction
2. vasodilatation
3. infarction
4. haemolysis
5. oedema

22.9 DNA synthesis is inhibited by:

1. prednisone
2. methane sulphonic acid
3. methotrexate
4. azathioprine
5. chloramphenicol

17.5 The production of red blood cells is depressed by the following conditions:

1. Chronic renal failure
2. Excessive administration of glucocorticoids
3. Subacute rheumatic fever
4. Myxoedema
5. Disseminated breast cancer

1.4 Post menopausal ovarian atrophy is associated with the following structural changes:

1. Stromal hyperplasia
2. Loss of ovarian weight
3. A proportionate decrease in size of the medulla
4. Disappearance of primordial follicles
5. Persistence of the germinal epithelium

4.1 Infection within a hospital may be:

1. dust-borne
2. water-borne
3. food-borne
4. hand-borne
5. endogenous

17.26 Disorders of clotting occur in association with:

1. vitamin A deficiency
2. vitamin K deficiency
3. hereditary angioneurotic oedema
4. haemophilia
5. obstructive jaundice

1.2 Hypertrophy is associated with:

1. an increase in the number of visible mitoses
2. an increase in the bulk of a tissue
3. an increase in the number of cells in an organ or tissue
4. an absolute decrease in interstitial tissue
5. an increase in functional capacity

16.9 Coarctation of the aorta is associated with:

1. a primary developmental anomaly of the third left aortic arch
2. the development of a collateral circulation to overcome the effects of the stenosis
3. strong femoral pulses
4. hypertension
5. erosion of the upper borders of the ribs

15.10 The following diseases are caused by chlamydia:

1. Yellow fever
2. Lymphogranuloma venereum
3. Mumps
4. Psittacosis
5. Herpes simplex

17.9 Congenital spherocytosis is a haemolytic disorder:

1. inherited as an autosomal recessive
2. associated with chronic anaemia
3. basically caused by a developmental defect of the red cell membrane
4. associated with massive enlargement of the spleen
5. in which the osmotic fragility of the red cell is diminished

21.3 The following refer to blood group antigens:

1. Lewis
2. Von Willebrand
3. Duffy
4. Turner
5. Kidd

5.6 Benzyl penicillin is:

1. bacteriostatic
2. destroyed by the enzyme penicillinase
3. insoluble in water
4. damaging to the nucleus of the bacterial cell
5. active against some viruses

21.8 The following antibodies may pass across the placenta:

1. Anti A isohaemagglutinin
2. Immune antiblood group A
3. Anti D (Rhesus)
4. Diphtheria antitoxin
5. Rheumatoid factor

Question number			Answer		
19.1	1. T	2. T	3. T	4. T	5. T
14.8	1. T	2. F	3. T	4. F	5. T
7.20	1. T	2. F	3. T	4. F	5. F
23.8	1. T	2. F	3. T	4. F	5. F
8.2	1. F	2. T	3. T	4. F	5. F
2.5	1. T	2. F	3. T	4. F	5. F
13.8	1. T	2. F	3. T	4. T	5. T
2.3	1. T	2. T	3. F	4. F	5. T
22.9	1. F	2. T	3. T	4. T	5. F
17.5	1. T	2. F	3. T	4. T	5. T
1.4	1. T	2. T	3. F	4. T	5. T
4.1	1. T	2. T	3. T	4. T	5. T
17.26	1. F	2. T	3. T	4. T	5. T
1.2	1. F	2. T	3. F	4. F	5. T
16.9	1. F	2. T	3. F	4. F	5. F
15.10	1. F	2. T	3. F	4. T	5. F
17.9	1. F	2. T	3. T	4. F	5. F
21.3	1. T	2. F	3. T	4. F	5. T
5.6	1. F	2. T	3. F	4. F	5. F
21.8	1. F	2. T	3. T	4. T	5. F

23.11 The glycogen storage diseases are associated with the following enzyme defects:

1. Amylase
2. Glucose-6-phosphatase
3. Amylo, 1, 6-glycosidase
4. Glutamic oxaloacetic transaminase
5. Nucleotide adenophosphodehydrogenase

4.13 The common pathogenic pyogenic organisms affecting man include:

1. *Staphylococcus aureus*
2. *Clostridium tetani*
3. *Staphylococcus albus*
4. *Bacteroides*
5. *Pseudomonas aeruginosa*

17.24 The chief characteristics of Burkitt's lymphoma are that:

1. it is commonest in young adults
2. it is associated with the Epstein Barr virus
3. it is uncommon in malarial areas
4. the commonest parts of the body involved are the facial bones and lower jaw
5. the characteristic cells of the tumour are poorly differentiated large lymphocytes and large pale histocytes

7.25 The following tests are based upon the delayed hypersensitivity reaction:

1. Schick test
2. Pseudo-Schick test
3. Frei test
4. Leishmanin test
5. Prausnitz-Kustner reaction

17.8 The following haemolytic disorders are congenital:

1. Thalassaemia
2. March haemoglobinuria
3. Microangiopathic haemolytic anaemia
4. Ovalocytosis
5. G6PD deficiency

9.2 Hypercalcaemia is associated with:

1. increased excitability of the neuromuscular apparatus
2. band keratitis
3. metastatic calcification
4. prolonged Q–T interval
5. renal stones

17.27 The formation of a clot is affected by the following substances:

1. Zinc
2. Calcium
3. Factor B
4. Factor IX
5. Kallikrein

12.10 The following biochemical disturbances occur in fulminating hepatic failure:

1. Metabolic acidosis
2. Hyperkalaemia
3. Hypoglycaemia
4. Fall in PO_2
5. Hypernatraemia

8.1 The total plasma protein level is low in:

1. patients suffering from protein losing entero-pathy
2. patients suffering from cardiac failure associated with oedema
3. oedema due to nephrotic syndrome
4. nutritional oedema
5. patients suffering from chronic liver disease

17.30 Which of the following functions are carried out by platelets:

1. Binding of antigen-antibody complexes
2. Secretion of clotting factors
3. Secretion of prostaglandins
4. Release of the Hageman factor
5. Release of vasoactive amines

23.13 Prostaglandins are:

1. formed from complement
2. vasodilators
3. involved in clotting
4. inhibited by azathioprine
5. inhibited by aspirin

17.21 Monocytic leukaemia:

1. is the commonest form of leukaemia
2. is associated with monocytes or monoblasts in the peripheral blood
3. may present with increasing anaemia
4. is associated with nodular infiltrative skin lesions
5. can present as an acute myelo-monocytic form

4.3 The following diseases are the result of arthropod-borne blood infections:

1. Cholera
2. Trypanosomiasis
3. Tetanus
4. Malaria
5. Hydatid disease

21.2 The following tests should be performed on donor blood before it is used for transfusion:

1. HbsAg
2. Van den Bergh
3. Wassermann test or the VDRL flocculation test
4. Acid phosphatase
5. Malaria smear

23.12 A vaccine:

1. contains one or more antigens
2. produces active immunity
3. contains one or more antibodies
4. stimulates polymorphonuclear leucocyte activity
5. can be administered orally

4.12 Staphylococci pathogenic to man:

1. produce a capsular polysaccharide
2. grow in irregular clusters in culture
3. produce coagulase
4. are resistant to penicillin
5. all produce an enterotoxin

17.23 Hodgkin's lymphoma has recently been re-classified into four histological groups. Regardless of classification, however, which of the following cell types are found in the lymph nodes in this disease?

1. Lymphocytes
2. Basophils
3. Eosinophils
4. Reed–Sternberg cells
5. Polymorphonuclear leucocytes

13.9 An enhancement of tumour growth or an increased incidence of tumour formation may occur:

1. following the long term administration of immunosuppressive drugs
2. following immunological enhancement
3. due to the release of soluble antigens by the tumour cells
4. due to an alteration of T-cell function
5. due to the excessive production or release of lysosomal enzymes

17.4 Iron deficiency anaemia may be associated with the following:

1. A sensitive and painful glossitis
2. Dysphagia
3. A rise in the liver iron
4. Koilonychia
5. Chlorosis

21.5 The physical results of Rhesus incompatibility include the following:

1. Hydrops fetalis
2. Hutchinson's teeth
3. Icterus neonatorum
4. Hepato-lenticular degeneration
5. Kernicterus

Question number	Answer				
23.11	1. F	2. T	3. T	4. F	5. F
4.13	1. T	2. F	3. F	4. T	5. T
17.24	1. F	2. T	3. F	4. T	5. T
7.25	1. F	2. T	3. T	4. T	5. F
17.8	1. T	2. F	3. F	4. T	5. T
9.2	1. F	2. T	3. T	4. F	5. T
17.27	1. F	2. T	3. F	4. T	5. F
12.10	1. F	2. F	3. T	4. T	5. F
8.1	1. T	2. F	3. T	4. T	5. T
17.30	1. T	2. F	3. T	4. F	5. T
23.13	1. F	2. T	3. T	4. F	5. T
17.21	1. F	2. T	3. T	4. T	5. T
4.3	1. F	2. T	3. F	4. T	5. F
21.2	1. T	2. F	3. T	4. F	5. T
23.12	1. T	2. T	3. F	4. F	5. T
4.12	1. F	2. T	3. T	4. T	5. F
17.23	1. T	2. F	3. T	4. T	5. T
13.9	1. T	2. T	3. T	4. T	5. F
17.4	1. F	2. T	3. F	4. T	5. T
21.5	1. T	2. F	3. T	4. F	5. T

17.15 An absolute lymphocytosis occurs in the following conditions:

1. Extensive skin diseases such as psoriasis, eczema, pemphigus
2. Loeffler's syndrome
3. Tuberculosis
4. Pertussis
5. Chronic lymphatic leukaemia

4.11 Renal tract infection is caused by a variety of bacteria including:

1. *Streptococcus pyogenes*
2. *Klebsiella pneumoniae*
3. *Streptococcus faecalis*
4. *Staphylococcus aureus*
5. *Escherichia coli*

8.3 Secondary hypogammaglobulinaemia occurs in:

1. sarcoidosis
2. congestive cardiac failure
3. malnutrition
4. protein losing enteropathy
5. nephrotic syndrome

12.5 A diminution in the bile salt pool and hence a diminished concentration of bile salts in the bile occurs:

1. in jejunal diverticulosis
2. in diseases affecting the terminal ileum such as Crohn's disease
3. due to the eating of refined carbohydrates
4. in ulcerative colitis
5. in congenital deficiency of cholesterol 7α-hydroxylase

17.1 A low mean corpuscular haemoglobin concentration occurs in the following:

1. Iron deficiency anaemia
2. Pernicious anaemia
3. The anaemia associated with infestation with the fish tapeworm *Diphyllobothrium latum*
4. The anaemia following extensive gastric resection
5. Sideroblastic anaemia

18.2 Increased amounts of erythropoietin are found in the plasma:

1. in pernicious anaemia
2. in iron deficiency anaemia
3. following bleeding
4. in erythroblastosis foetalis
5. in Kwashiorkor

17.3 The presence of Hb-A$_2$ (α^2 δ^2) in the red corpuscles is associated with:

1. increased osmotic resistance of the red cells
2. reduced life span of the red corpuscles
3. congenital spherocytosis
4. thalassaemia
5. sickle-cell anaemia

4.4 *Streptococcus faecalis*:

1. is a common inhabitant of the gastrointestinal tract
2. grows in long chains
3. flourishes in bile-salt lactose media
4. is concerned in the aetiology of periodontal disease
5. is an opportunistic rather than a true pathogen

13.11 The incidence of tumours is increased in:

1. sarcoidosis
2. Wiskott Aldrich syndrome
3. ataxia telangiectasis
4. patients treated over long periods with cortico-steroids
5. patients receiving azathioprine

17.17 Myeloid metaplasia may be associated with:

1. a variable peripheral white count
2. extramedullary haemopoiesis
3. the Philadelphia chromosome
4. a decreased number of megakaryocytes in the marrow
5. anaemia

14.11 The 'doubling time' of a malignant tumour is affected by a number of factors including:

1. tumour necrosis
2. exfoliation
3. the percentage of cells in the resting phase
4. the oxygen content of the tumour cells environment
5. nuclear size

17.16 Acute myeloblastic leukaemia:

1. is most common in young adults
2. is associated with the presence of a large number of primitive cells in the marrow and peripheral blood
3. is associated with peripheral white counts in excess of 100 000 per μl
4. may be associated with a normal white count
5. marrow aspirates show decreased cellularity

8.4 A monoclonal gammopathy occurs in the following diseases:

1. Lepromatous leprosy
2. Kala-azar
3. Multiple myeloma
4. Lymphatic leukaemia
5. Active chronic hepatitis

11.4 Idiopathic haemochromatosis is associated with:

1. an excessive production of melanin
2. decreased absorption of iron from the gut
3. the deposition of haemosiderin in the liver
4. diabetes
5. females

13.3 The following pathological conditions can be regarded as precancerous:

1. Paget's disease of bone
2. Leukoplakia
3. Fibroadenosis of the breast
4. Duodenal ulceration
5. Cervical erosions

16.7 The investigations performed in a patient suffering from Raynaud's phenomenon should include:

1. assay of haemagglutinating antibodies
2. rheumatoid factor
3. antimitochondrial antibodies
4. serum potassium
5. X-ray of the root of the neck

10.1 Oedema occurs in:

1. Cushing's syndrome
2. primary aldosteronism
3. Zollinger–Ellison syndrome
4. Klinefelter's syndrome
5. pregnancy

14.2 Broder's classification of tumours attempted to classify tumours according to:

1. their origin
2. the degree of differentiation of a tumour
3. the degree of stromal response
4. the degree of lymphocytic infiltration of the tumour
5. the number of mitoses found in a given area of the tumour

16.13 A myocardial infarct may be associated with:

1. hypotension
2. a fall in the plasma GOT
3. endocardial thrombosis
4. a red infarct
5. atrial rather than ventricular fibrillation

15.9 Interferon:

1. is a complement component
2. may be induced by bacterial endotoxin
3. may be induced by Poly I:C
4. is a dialysable factor
5. is species-specific

11.3 The following endocrine abnormalities lead to generalized pigmentation:

1. Cushing's disease
2. Carcinoid tumours
3. Zollinger–Ellison syndrome
4. Addison's disease
5. Sheehan's syndrome

Question number		Answer			
17.15	1. F	2. F	3. T	4. T	5. T
4.11	1. F	2. T	3. T	4. T	5. T
8.3	1. F	2. F	3. T	4. T	5. T
12.5	1. F	2. T	3. T	4. F	5. T
17.1	1. T	2. F	3. F	4. T	5. F
18.2	1. T	2. T	3. T	4. T	5. F
17.3	1. T	2. T	3. F	4. T	5. F
4.4	1. T	2. F	3. T	4. T	5. T
13.11	1. F	2. T	3. T	4. F	5. T
17.17	1. T	2. T	3. F	4. F	5. T
14.11	1. T	2. T	3. T	4. T	5. F
17.16	1. F	2. T	3. F	4. T	5. F
8.4	1. F	2. F	3. T	4. T	5. F
11.4	1. T	2. F	3. T	4. T	5. F
13.3	1. T	2. T	3. F	4. F	5. F
16.7	1. T	2. T	3. F	4. F	5. T
10.1	1. T	2. F	3. T	4. F	5. F
14.2	1. F	2. T	3. F	4. F	5. T
16.13	1. T	2. F	3. T	4. F	5. F
15.9	1. F	2. T	3. T	4. F	5. T
11.3	1. T	2. F	3. F	4. T	5. F

Part 2: Questions and answers with explanations

Section 1. HYPERTROPHY

1.1 Disuse atrophy follows:

1. blockage of the duct of an exocrine gland
2. immobilisation of a joint
3. interference with the nerve supply to the muscles controlling joint movement
4. interference with the blood supply
5. the diminished secretion of trophic hormones

1. True
An excellent example is the pancreas. Ligation of the main pancreatic duct leads to atrophy of the exocrine portion of the gland but the endocrine portion, i.e. islets of Langerhans, continue to function normally.

2. True
Immobilisation of the knee provides a good example. An internal derangement of this joint, such as damage to a cartilage, is rapidly followed by atrophy of the quadriceps group of muscles.

3. False
Interruption of the nerve supply to a group of muscles causes a specific neuropathic atrophy in the affected group of muscles. However, the bone to which such muscles are attached may undergo true atrophy due simply to inactivity if the condition is irreversible, e.g. anterior poliomyelitis.

4. False
Interference with the blood supply to a tissue causes atrophy due to defective nutrition.

5. False
The diminished secretion of trophic hormones such as T_4 by the thyroid does produce atrophic changes

in target organs such as the skin, hair follicles, sweat gland and sebaceous glands but this is not disuse atrophy. These changes can be readily reversed by the administration of thyroxine.

1.2 Hypertrophy is associated with:

1. an increase in the number of visible mitoses
2. an increase in the bulk of a tissue
3. an increase in the number of cells in an organ or tissue
4. an absolute decrease in interstitial tissue
5. an increase in functional capacity

1. False
In pure hypertrophy the number of cells remains the same in contrast to hyperplasia in which the number of cells increases. No evidence of excessive mitoses is, therefore, normally seen.

2. True
This is the chief change in hypertrophy. It is seen to best advantage in the hypertrophied muscles of an athlete or in the cardiac muscle in response to hypertension or aortic stenosis or regurgitation.

3. False
Pure hypertrophy is not associated with an increase in the number of cells but only with an increase in the size of those already present.

4. False
The volume of interstitial tissue does not alter. Any apparent decrease is relative, produced by the enlargement of the specialised cells of the organ or tissue.

5. True
The functional capacity of all organs and tissues in which hypertrophy occurs is increased. For example, the increased thickness and length of hypertrophied muscles leads to increased power. Another example is the hypertrophy of the remaining kidney following unilateral nephrectomy. The remaining kidney, if this is normal, increases in size and functional capacity. In part this is due to true hypertrophy but in addition hyperplasia also occurs with an increase

in the number of component cells of the glomeruli and tubules.

1.3 Old age is specifically associated with atrophic changes in:

1. bone
2. the kidneys
3. the bone marrow
4. the brain
5. the ovaries

1. True
The radiological density of bone progressively decreases in both men and women with advancing age. This change is indistinguishable from osteoporosis, in which condition the amount of uncalcified bone may become so great that bone pain and fractures may occur.

2. True
Increasing age is associated with a gradual loss in the number of nephrons and a gradual reduction in renal functional capacity. At ninety years of age the overall function of kidneys has diminished by about 50 per cent. The diminution of glomerular filtration is particularly important in relation to the administration of drugs such as digitalis and some antibiotics.

3. True
Gradual replacement of the red marrow takes place with advancing age.

4. True
Old age is associated with loss of neurones and neuroglial overgrowth causing senile or presenile dementia. These changes occur more rapidly in the presence of ischaemia.

5. True
Ovarian atrophy is associated with a decline in weight of these organs from approximately 14 g to around 5 g in the sixth decade. The primordial follicles largely disappear and marked stromal hyperplasia occurs.

1.4 Post menopausal ovarian atrophy is associated with the following structural changes:

1. Stromal hyperplasia

2. Loss of ovarian weight
3. A proportionate decrease in size of the medulla
4. Disappearance of primordial follicles
5. Persistence of the germinal epithelium

1. True
Marked stromal hyperplasia occurs after 40 years of age, possibly due to continued hormone production by the ovaries.

2. True
The weight of the premenopausal ovary is about 14 g, by the seventh decade this falls to 5 g.

3. False
Relative to the cortex the medullary portion of the ovary, in which the corpora albicantia and candicantia are situated, is proportionately larger in the post menopausal ovary.

4. True
Rarely a few immature follicles undergoing maturation and atresia may be seen in the corticomedullary junction in the first five years after the menopause.

5. True
The germinal epithelium persists and follows the various convolutions on the surface but in some places, however, this intimate connection with the surface may be lost and small cysts may form.

1.5 Starvation is associated with a reduction in size of the:

1. fat depots
2. heart
3. central nervous system
4. liver
5. bones

In the first phase of starvation the fat depots disappear and this is later followed by a gradual reduction in the size of organs such as the gastrointestinal tract, liver and heart while the central nervous system and skeleton remain unaffected. The correct answers are, therefore,

1. True

2. True
3. False
4. True
5. False

An exception to this general pattern occurs in kwashiorkor. In this condition, which affects infants and young children in many parts of Southern and Central Africa and the Far East, the diet is deficient in high grade protein but moderately adequate in total calories due to a high carbohydrate intake. Growth is impaired but the liver is enlarged, grossly fatty and depleted of protein and RNA.

1.6 Metaplasia, the transformation of one fully differentiated tissue into another, occurs in:

1. connective tissue elements
2. the gastrointestinal tract
3. the central nervous system
4. the biliary system
5. the urothelium

1. True
True bone may occasionally develop in an operation scar.

2. True
Metaplasia occurs in some parts of the gastrointestinal tract under abnormal circumstances. A common site is in the mucus secreting columnar epithelium of the anal canal. When this mucosa prolapses through the anal sphincter the resulting chronic irritation results in a change to squamous epithelium. Causes of prolapse include severe haemorrhoids and true prolapse.

3. False
No metaplastic changes occur in the central nervous system.

4. True
Metaplasia of the gall bladder epithelium is associated with the presence of gall stones. This may be eventually followed by the development of a squamous cell carcinoma because the original change is from tall columnar to a squamous type of epithelium.

5. True
Epithelial metaplasia is usually associated with a change to a less specialised or complex type of epithelium. The urothelium is an important exception. In the bladder the presence of chronic inflammation (excluding tuberculosis) leads to cystitis cystica. The transitional epithelium grows downwards in solid clumps into the submucosa and if these become detached a central space may develop and since these cells may acquire mucus-secreting properties the end result is a glandular mucous membrane. A similar process in the ureters lead to the condition of ureteritis cystitis. Calculi in the urinary tract cause the normal transitional epithelium to become squamous in type, a change which may be followed by the development of a squamous carcinoma.

Section 2. ACUTE INFLAMMATION

2.1 Acute inflammation can be caused by:

1. *Streptococcus pneumoniae*
2. *Mycobacterium tuberculosis*
3. *Neisseria meningitidis*
4. *Mycobacterium leprae*
5. *Borrelia vincenti*

1. True
Streptococcus pneumoniae is the causal organism of lobar pneumonia.

2. True
Although *Mycobacterium tuberculosis* is more commonly associated with 'chronic' inflammation acute tuberculous inflammation does occur particularly following infection of the meninges or pleura.

3. True
Neisseria meningitidis is the causal organism of acute meningitis. This disease was once referred to as 'spotted fever' because in the presence of meningococcal septicaemia a haemorrhagic rash occurs.

4. False
Mycobacterium leprae is never associated with acute inflammation. Two forms of leprosy occur, lepromatous and tuberculoid.

5. True
Borrelia vincenti is the causal agent of Vincent's angina, an acute inflammation of the gums or oropharynx. The organism itself is an anaerobic flexuous spirochaete with 3 to 8 irregular coils. It is a normal commensal in the mouth.

2.2 The following agents produce an acute inflammatory reaction in unsensitised individuals:

1. Lipopolysaccharide
2. Albumin
3. Ultraviolet light
4. Insulin
5. Carbon particles

1. True
Lipopolysaccharides are the chemical structure of bacterial endotoxins. An intradermal injection causes an immediate acute inflammatory reaction. A subsequent intravenous injection of polysaccharide 24 hours later will produce a local haemorrhagic reaction associated with tissue necrosis at the site of the previous intradermal injection. (Schwartzmann reaction)

2. False
An intradermal injection of albumin does not cause an inflammatory reaction unless an individual has been previously sensitised.

3. True
Radiation injury which may be due to heat or ionising radiation in addition to ultraviolet light can cause an acute inflammatory reaction. The initial reaction is the triple response which follows histamine release.

4. False
Insulin does not cause an inflammatory reaction in unsensitised individuals.

5. False
Carbon particles are biologically inactive although some of the carbon which is inhaled is engulfed by macrophages and is retained within the relatively immobile alveoli adjacent to the bronchioles, blood vessels and fibrous septa producing the blackening

which is seen in nearly every adult lung of city dwellers at autopsy.

2.3 Normally the features of acute inflammation include:

1. vasoconstriction
2. vasodilatation
3. infarction
4. haemolysis
5. oedema

1. True
The earliest change following the initiation of acute inflammation is constriction of small blood vessels.

2. True
The initial capillary constriction is rapidly followed by vasodilatation. This gives rise to the first part of the triple response described by Lewis, the 'red line'. This, in turn, is followed by arteriolar dilatation producing the 'flare' after which increased permeability of the small blood vessels causes the appearance of a 'wheal'. This triple response can be readily reproduced by pricking histamine into the skin and can be blocked by antihistamines. It is, however, probably of little practical importance in acute bacterial inflammation.

3. False
Infarction is commonly due to the obstruction of an end artery, usually by an embolus. This causes a segmental area of tissue necrosis and whilst the necrotic area itself does not become inflamed the surrounding tissues show all the histological changes associated with inflammation.

4. False
The intravascular lysis of erythrocytes does not normally accompany acute inflammation. It may, however, develop due to the liberation of exotoxins by the infecting organisms, such as *Clostridium welchii* and *Streptococcus pyogenes*.

5. True
The exudation of fluid from the blood vessels in an inflamed area gives rise to swelling which is one of

the cardinal signs of inflammation. The exudate is due to several factors, which include:

(a) the hydrostatic pressure in the small blood vessels exceeding the osmotic pressure of the plasma proteins
(b) an increase in small vessel permeability caused by the chemical mediators of inflammation
(c) an inability of the lymphatics to remove the increased quantities of interstitial fluid.

2.4 The blood flow through acutely inflamed tissues is decreased by the following events:

1. Increased cellular concentration in the blood flowing through the inflamed part
2. Loss of protein from the dilated capillaries
3. Aggregation of the red cells
4. Adherence of leucocytes to the capillary endothelium
5. Lewis' axon reflex

1. True
The cellular concentration of the blood in the capillaries and post-capillary venules of an inflamed tissue is increased. This occurs because fluid escapes from the dilated blood vessels because of their increased permeability, thus increasing the blood's viscosity.

2. False
Although protein loss does occur the fluid loss is greater. This leads to an elevation in the plasma protein concentration and hence an increase in viscosity.

3. True
The red cells aggregate into rouleaux which leads to sludging. A process first described by Kniseley. This further increases the viscosity of the blood.

4. True
The effective lumen of the post-capillary venules is greatly reduced by the adherence of the leucocytes to one another and to the endothelium of the capillaries and post-capillary venules.

5. False
It is doubtful whether the axon reflex is of any practical importance in the acute inflammatory process.

2.5 The magnitude of the exudate associated with acute inflammation depends upon:

1. changes in the endothelium of the capillaries and venules
2. lymphocyte activation
3. the osmotic pressure of the plasma proteins
4. the plasma Ca^{++} level
5. the plasma K^+ level

1. True
A number of chemical mediators act on the capillary endothelium to increase its permeability thus allowing the escape of protein rich fluid into the area of acute inflammation. Among these various chemicals are histamine, a variety of kinins, prostaglandins and a number of complement components.

2. False
There is no evidence that lymphocyte activation, which is important in cell-mediated immune reactions, delayed hypersensitivity and chronic inflammation, plays a major role in acute inflammation.

3. True
The osmotic pressure of the plasma and the inflammatory exudate is dependent upon the protein concentration. When the osmotic pressure in the exudate is higher than in the vessels, more fluid will be drawn into the exudate.

4. False
There is no evidence, as yet, that plasma Ca^{++} levels affect the acute inflammatory response although the concentration of calcium does, however, play an important role in intracellular events. Thus the movement of extracellular calcium into the cell can activate a number of events through cyclic nucleotides.

5. False
There is no evidence that potassium concentration plays any part in the local inflammatory response. Hypo- or hyperkalaemia does, however, have important physiological effects, particularly on the myocardium.

2.6 The following cell types are involved in acute inflammation:

1. Polymorphonuclear leucocytes

2. Lymphocytes
3. Endothelial cells
4. Epithelioid cells
5. Mast cells

1. True
The polymorphonuclear leucocyte is the chief cell in acute inflammation. It is attracted to the inflammatory focus by a variety of chemotactic factors among which the most important are the C3a and C5a complement components.

2. False
Lymphocytes play no major role in the early stages of acute inflammation. They are, however, of greater importance in chronic inflammation and are particularly important in those inflammatory processes which involve cell mediated immunity.

3. True
Changes in the endothelium result in an increase in capillary permeability and the adherence of polymorphonuclear leucocytes to the walls of small blood vessels. Such changes are probably brought about by chemical mediators among which histamine, bradykinin and the prostaglandins appear to be important.

4. False
Epithelioid cells are not seen in acute inflammatory conditions. They are derived from mononuclear phagocytic cells and are commonly seen in the centre of granulomas produced by agents such as *Mycobacterium tuberculosis* which usually causes long standing chronic inflammation.

5. True
Mast cells secrete histamine, serotonin, SRS-A and kallikrein, all of which play a role in the acute inflammatory process. Degranulation of the mast cells is an important step in the release of histamine from these cells, this chemical agent being one of the earliest chemical mediators found in acutely inflamed tissues.

2.7 The magnitude of leucocyte migration into an area infected with bacteria is governed by:

1. the type of organism causing the inflammatory lesion

2. chemotaxins
3. the C5a complement component
4. the phosphatase levels in the inflamed area
5. the formation of pus

1. True
The intensity of the leucocyte infiltration into an infected lesion varies considerably. Some bacteria, notably the pyogenic organisms, such as *Streptococcus pyogenes*, *Staphylococcus aureus* and *Streptococcus pneumoniae* are associated with an intense leucocytic infiltration. Others such as *Salmonella typhi* and *Clostridum welchii*, although a cause of severe inflammation, do not provoke such a severe degree of leucocytic infiltration.

2. True
Chemotaxins are chemical substances which simulate migration of the leucocytes in a particular direction. Identifiable chemotaxins include bacterial products, lysates of the polymorphonuclear cells and extracts from the inflamed tissues.

3. True
C5a is a product of reacted complement. In certain circumstances it can be shown that complement depletion is associated with a decrease in leucocyte migration into an inflamed area.

4. False
Phosphatase levels play no part in the acute inflammatory process.

5. True
Lysates of the polymorphonuclear cells are very potent chemotactic agents when incubated with serum and it can, therefore, be assumed that pus formation increases leucocyte migration.

2.8 The main components of the pyogenic membrane are:

1. eosinophils
2. capillary loops
3. hyaluronidase
4. polymorphonuclear leucocytes
5. fibroblasts

1. False
Eosinophil cells play no part in the acute inflammatory response which normally initiates the formation of a pyogenic membrane.

2. True
The proliferation of capillary loops is a characteristic feature of granulation tissue. When the original factor initiating the formation of the membrane, e.g. the pyogenic organism, has been eliminated either by the body's natural defence mechanisms or by the administration of antibiotics the capillary loops grow into the inflamed zone at up to 2 mm a day supported by ground substance.

3. False
Hyaluronidase is an enzyme produced by some bacteria such as the clostridia which are responsible for gas gangrene. This enables the organisms to spread through the tissue planes.

4. True
Polymorphonuclear leucocytes migrate into the ground substance from the capillary loop in order to phagocytose bacteria. Peripheral to these cells may be plasma cells, lymphocytes and macrophages, all cells concerned with the natural defence mechanisms.

5. True
Fibroblasts accompany the capillary loops and are dependent upon them for their oxygen supply. When the stage of healing has been reached the fibroblasts lay down collagen.

2.9 The following are the chemical mediators involved in acute inflammation:

1. Complement
2. Histamine
3. Insulin
4. Bradykinin
5. Lymphokine

1. True
The C3a and C5a components of complement are powerful chemotactic agents attracting polymorphonuclear leucocytes to a site of acute inflammation. In

addition these compounds also act as anaphylatoxins causing histamine release from the mast cells with the result that plain muscle contracts and vasoconstriction follows.

2. True
Histamine liberated by the degranulation of mast cells is one of the most important causes of the changes seen in the early phase of acute inflammation, a phase which can be markedly depressed by the administration of antihistamines.

3. False
This substance plays no known role in acute inflammation. It is secreted by the β cells of the islets of Langerhans and is a major factor in controlling the circulating level of glucose. An increase in its secretion causes an enhanced uptake of glucose by the hepatocytes and a decrease in glucose absorption from the intestine.

4. True
Bradykinin is a nonapeptide derived from a plasma euglobulin by the digestion of the latter by proteolytic enzymes. Among these are kallikrein which is present in the plasma as an inactive precursor which is activated by the Hageman factor. Bradykinin causes pain, erythema and increased venular permeability and hence swelling of an acutely inflamed area.

5. False
Lymphokines are not concerned with acute inflammation but are considered to be the mediators of delayed hypersensitivity. They are secreted by lymphocytes which have been activated by a specific antigen or mitogen. They are chemotactic to mononuclear cells, inhibit the migration of macrophages *in vitro* and cause delayed inflammatory reactions in the skin.

2.10 The following substances are involved in acute inflammation:

1. Peptides
2. Lectins
3. Plasmin
4. LATS
5. PGE_1

1. True

Peptides composed of between 8 and 14 amino acid residues increase vascular permeability and hence increase the volume of exudate accompanying an acute inflammatory reaction. Such peptides are derived from protein in the exudate due to the action of proteolytic enzymes derived from the plasma, tissue cells and polymorphonuclear leucocytes.

2. False

Lectins play no part in acute inflammation. They are proteins derived from plants which act as mitogens, i.e. induce mitosis or cause lymphocyte transformation in lymphocytes. Among these compounds are phytohaemagglutinin (PHA), concanavalin A (ConA) and Pokeweed mitogen.

3. True

Plasmin is intimately concerned with the acute inflammatory response. It is a proteolytic enzyme produced from the plasma plasminogen by the action of the enzyme kallikrein. Among its various actions plasmin breaks down fibrin, splits kininogen to form bradykinin and acts on the C3 component of complement to produce C3a and C3b. The former is a strong chemotactic agent and anaphylatoxin and the latter promotes phagocytosis.

4. False

LATS, long acting thyroid stimulator is not involved in acute inflammation.

5. True

This substance causes vasodilatation, increases capillary permeability and potentiates the activity of kinins. It, therefore, plays an important role in acute inflammation. PGE_1 is formed from the substrate arachadonic acid, the inhibition of its activity by aspirin and indomethacin is considered to be the basis of the anti-inflammatory activity of these compounds.

2.11 Phagocytosis is promoted by:

1. hyaluronidase
2. neuraminidase
3. the hexose monophosphate shunt
4. immunoglobulin
5. complement

1. False
Hyaluronidase plays no part in phagocytosis. It is, however, an important factor in the spread of infections caused by the clostridia, staphylococci and streptococci which secrete this enzyme. Its action is to break down hyaluronic acid which is a normal constituent of intercellular ground substance.

2. False
Neuraminidase plays no part in phagocytosis. This substance is an enzyme produced by certain viruses and bacteria which splits a chemical bond between neuraminic acid and other sugars. Neuraminic acid is an important structural component of the surface glycoproteins of many cells.

3. False
The hexose monophosphate shunt does not promote phagocytosis but it is a significant factor in causing the death of micro-organisms following phagocytosis. This shunt is a powerful system of enzymes present in polymorphonuclear leucocytes and macrophages. It involves the activation of NADH and NADPH oxidases leading to the formation of powerful oxidising agents including hydrogen peroxide.

4. True
Specific antibodies are important agents in the opsonisation of bacteria prior to phagocytosis.

5. True
Complement components have an action which was known in the past as non-specific opsonisation. The conversion of C3 through either the classical or alternative pathway leads to the formation of C3b. This is recognised by specific cell receptors, by a process of immune adherence, leading to phagocytosis.

2.12 Micro-organisms which have undergone phagocytosis are killed by:

1. lecithinase
2. lysozyme
3. lysosomal enzymes
4. lymphokine
5. hydrogen peroxide

1. False
This enzyme has no action on micro-organisms. It is one of the many enzymes produced by the clostridia, its specific action is to haemolyse the erythrocytes by attacking their cell membranes.

2. True
This enzyme, which is found in the polymorphonuclear leucocytes and at many other sites including tears, plays an important role in the destruction of micro-organisms. It acts by destroying muramic acid which is one of the chief constituents of the cell wall of bacteria.

3. True
The lysosomal enzymes are a group of proteolytic and hydrolytic enzymes capable of digesting ingested micro-organisms. High concentrations of these enzymes are secreted around ingested bacteria following fusion of lysosomes with the phagosome.

4. False
Lymphokines play no direct part in the destruction of ingested micro-organisms. However, these substances do activate the macrophages causing the increased production of lysosomal enzymes. Lymphokines are produced by the action of specific antigens or mitogens on primed T-lymphocytes. They are important in the body's defence against certain micro-organisms and are concerned with delayed hypersensitivity reactions.

5. True
The intracellular release of peroxides including H_2O_2 plays a large part in the destruction of ingested micro-organisms. These substances are produced as a side product of the hexose monophosphate shunt which acts through NADH and NADPH oxidases.

2.13 Pus contains:

1. lipids
2. fibrin
3. collagen
4. plasma cells
5. polymorphonuclear leucocytes

1. True

Lipids are present in pus. They are derived from the plasma lipoproteins and from cellular breakdown products. Cholesterol may be found in old pus.

2. True

Pus contains fibrin because the activation of the coagulation system by the Hageman factor converts plasma fibrinogen into fibrin. The Hageman factor, Factor XII in the international classification of plasma coagulation factors, may be activated by kallikrein.

3. False

Collagen is not a constituent of pus although its breakdown products may be present due to the activity of enzymes known as collagenases. During healing collagen is laid down by fibroblasts.

4. False

Plasma cells are not normally found in the pus formed as a result of acute inflammation. Chiefly they are found, together with lymphocytes, in the lymph nodes, spleen and gut but they are also present in the organised granulomas which form in "chronic inflammatory" lesions such as those which develop in rheumatoid arthritis.

5. True

The major cellular component of pus consists of dead or living polymorphonuclear leucocytes. These cells, when living, cause local tissue breakdown and the destruction of micro-organisms, if these are the cause of the acute inflammatory process, because of their high content of lysosomal enzymes and their phagocytic activity. Polymorphonuclear leucocytes are attracted to the site of an acute inflammatory reaction by a variety of chemotactic agents, one of the most potent of which *in vitro* is a lysate of the polymorphonuclear leucocytes themselves.

2.14 Septicaemia is associated with:

1. bacteraemia
2. toxaemia
3. the multiplication of bacteria in the blood stream
4. invasion of the blood stream by organisms multiplying elsewhere in the circulation, e.g. the peritoneum
5. multiple haemorrhagic foci in the tissues

1. False
The term bacteraemia implies that bacteria are circulating but not multiplying in the blood stream. Nevertheless, a bacteraemia can be dangerous because any bacteria in the blood stream may settle in various parts of the body. For example, osteomyelitis in children is believed to follow bacteraemia, the responsible organism, commonly the *Staphylococcus aureus*, being deposited in the metaphysis of the long bones.

2. True
Profound toxaemia with high fever complicates a septicaemia because of the toxins liberated from the responsible bacteria. These are pyrogenic themselves and also cause the formation of pyrogens due to tissue damage.

3. True
The essential feature of a septicaemia is the multiplication of bacteria in the blood stream. An example is infection by the plague bacillus, *Yersinia pestis*.

4. False
In patients suffering from severe peritonitis caused by *Escherichia coli* the organisms in the blood stream are probably invaders from the inflamed peritoneal cavity.

5. True
Small haemorrhages commonly occur in various organs and tissues. These are caused either by the effects of the accompanying toxaemia on the endothelium or by metastatic foci of bacterial growth.

Section 3. CHRONIC INFLAMMATION AND GRANULOMA FORMATION

3.1 Necrosis occurs as a concomitant feature of chronic inflammation in:

1. leprosy
2. tuberculosis
3. syphilis
4. actinomycosis
5. coccidiomycosis

1. False

Necrosis is an inconspicuous feature of both the epithelioid cell granuloma of tuberculoid leprosy and the aggregates of macrophages containing huge numbers of lepra bacilli which constitute the essential lesion of lepromatous leprosy. Tissue injury in the latter is probably mainly due to pressure. In the former necrosis is rare and leprosy bacilli are often difficult to find.

2. True

The characteristic central caseous area of the typical tubercle caused by the *Mycobacterium tuberculosis* is due to necrosis. Caseous material contains a high content of lipid and frequently a large number of bacilli. Aggregation of the follicles finally leads to the development of a tuberculous abscess and if liquefaction of the caseous material occurs the abscess begins to track through or along tissue planes forming the typical collar stud or psoas abscess.

3. True

Coagulative necrosis and caseation is typical of the gumma formed in tertiary syphilis. How the necrosis is brought about remains doubtful but it may be due to ischaemia caused by the associated endarteritis obliterans.

4. True

Necrosis is typical of an advanced actinomycotic lesion caused by the *Actinomyces bovis*, a bacterium related to the mycobacteria. The centre of an actinomycotic lesion contains pus in which are found the 'sulphur granules' which are grey-yellow in colour formed by colonies of filaments resembling fungal mycelia.

5. True

Coccidiomycosis is a fungal infection. The pulmonary lesion is morphologically similar to that of tuberculosis accompanied by central necrosis and micro-abscesses. These lesions frequently become calcified. Healing is associated with the development of a positive coccidioidin delayed hypersensitivity skin reaction.

3.2 The following belong to the mononuclear phagocyte system:

1. Macrophages

2. Mast cells
3. Epithelioid cells
4. Fibroblasts
5. Küpffer cells

1. True
The macrophage is the prototype of the cells belonging to the mononuclear phagocyte system. One of the most important characteristics of this cell which was first described by Metchnikoff is its ability to phagocytose foreign particulate and colloidal particles, but they are also important in processing antigen for lymphocyte recognition. It is the active non-specific effector cell in cell-mediated immunity and in host resistance to infection by facultative and obligate intracellular micro-organisms, e.g. mycobacteria, protozoa and viruses. Macrophages are derived from bone marrow precursors via circulating monocytes and they are easily recognised histologically by observing their uptake of carbon particles.

2. False
Mast cells are not a part of the MPS. They are the effector cells of IgE induced allergic reactions. Degranulated by antigen-antibody complexes they release histamine and other vasoactive substances such as serotonin and SRS-A.

3. True
Epithelioid cells represent an activated form of the cells of the MPS, they are, however, poorly phagocytic but possess intense enzymatic activity. Such cells are found in the centre of immunologically induced tuberculoid-type granulomas and they may aggregate to form the Langhans type of giant cell.

4. False
Fibroblasts are not related to the mononuclear phagocyte system although they may be found in close proximity to macrophages and epithelioid cells in granulomas. The function of fibroblasts is to secrete collagen.

5. True
Küpffer cells are derived from precursor cells in the bone marrow that circulate as monocytes and then settle in the sinuses of the liver forming actively phagocytic cells.

3.3 Malignant disease may complicate the following chronic inflammatory diseases:

1. Chronic osteomyelitis
2. Sarcoidosis
3. Asbestosis
4. Schistosomiasis
5. Ulcerative colitis

1. True
Although extremely rare squamous cell cancers were once seen in and around the skin sinuses associated with chronic osteomyelitis. The present rarity of the condition is due to the more effective treatment of osteomyelitis in the acute stage. The incidence of chronic osteomyelitis with the development of a large involucrum and chronically draining sinuses is extremely low in the Western World.

2. False
Sarcoidosis is not associated with malignant change.

3. True
Asbestosis is associated with the development of both squamous cell carcinoma and mesothelioma, 60 per cent of the latter being due to exposure to asbestos, this relationship being first noted in South Africa. The fibre type associated with mesothelioma is crocidolite and the latent interval between exposure and the development of the tumour itself may be as long as 40 years. Such tumours are not necessarily associated with pulmonary fibrosis.

4. True
This disease is due to infestation with the dioecious trematodes, *Schistosoma haematobium*, *mansoni* and *japonicum*. In Egypt the predominant infection is with *S. haematobium* and the adult parasites lie in the veins of the bladder. The eggs laid by the female pass into the submucosa and excite a granulomatous reaction which is later followed by metaplasia of the transitional cell urothelium to a squamous type. Squamous cell carcinoma then develops in a proportion of the victims, particularly infected Egyptians.

5. True
It is now well recognised that ulcerative colitis is a 'premalignant condition'. The incidence of malig-

nancy increases with the duration and totality of the disease being rarely seen in its more distal forms. At least one third of all cases with a history longer than 12 years develop cancer, usually multifocally.

3.4 Accumulation of macrophages is a prominent histological feature of the lesions produced by the following diseases:

1. Leishmaniasis
2. Extrinsic allergic alveolitis
3. Gaucher's disease
4. Legionnaire's disease
5. Letterer–Siwe's disease

1. True
Both cutaneous leishmaniasis (oriental sore) and systemic leishmaniasis (kala-azar) are associated with lesions in which a particular feature is the large number of macrophages present. These contain the Leishman–Donovan bodies which are the amastigote form of the parasite.

2. False
One example of extrinsic allergic alveolitis is Farmer's lung which is caused by the inhalation of the spores of *Micropolyspora faeni* found in mouldy hay. The lesion is caused by the deposition of immune complexes which activate complement giving rise to pulmonary fibrosis.

3. True
One of the chief features of Gaucher's disease which is caused by a deficiency of the enzyme glucocerebrosidase is a massive accumulation of macrophages in the spleen and to a lesser extent in the liver and lymph nodes. These become distended with the lipid glucocerebroside due to the enzyme defect.

4. False
A severe form of pyogenic bronchopneumonia with an almost lobar distribution. The disease occurs in epidemics and is believed to be caused by a Gram-negative bacillus, *Legionella*.

5. True
A form of 'Histiocytosis X' which is a term applied to

three conditions, Letterer–Siwe's disease, Hand–Schüller–Christian disease and eosinophil granuloma of bone. The condition referred to occurs in infancy and early childhood and runs a rapidly fatal course. It is characterised by hepatosplenomegaly, lymphadenopathy and multiple nodules in the skin and bone marrow. The affected organs show massive replacement by proliferated macrophage-like cells which are swollen, pale and contain phagocytosed debris.

3.5 Hyperplasia of the lymphoid tissue is a prominent feature in the following conditions:

1. Toxoplasmosis
2. Leishmaniasis
3. Chronic dermatitis
4. Silicosis
5. Berylliosis

1. True
Lymph node enlargement, caused chiefly by a reactive hyperplasia of all components of the node, is a prominent feature of toxoplasmosis, caused by infection with the protozoan, *Toxoplasma gondii*. In addition the germinal centres are larger than those observed in similar infections.

2. False
Specific hyperplasia of the lymphoid tissues does not occur in cutaneous leishmaniasis, otherwise known as oriental sore, caused by the protozoan, *Leishmania tropica*. In the systemic form of the disease, kala-azar caused by *Leishmania donovani*, hepatosplenomegaly occurs due to collections of macrophages which contain the Leishman–Donovan bodies. The latter are parasitic amastigotes.

3. True
Chronic dermatitis is associated with dermatopathic lymphadenopathy in which there may be replacement of paracortical areas with macrophages and enlargement of the germinal centres.

4. False
Silicosis does not appear to affect lymphoid tissue

except to cause fibrosis. Fibrosis of inguinal lymphoid tissue is thought to be a cause of non-filarial elephantiasis in Ethiopia, as a result of absorption of silica through the skin.

5. False
Beryllium causes fibrosis of the lung when inhaled. It is also a contact sensitiser. It does not seem particularly to affect lymphoid tissue.

3.6 Giant cells are characteristically found in the pathological lesions associated with the following diseases:

1. Actinomycosis
2. Schistosomiasis
3. Primary biliary cirrhosis
4. Lepromatous leprosy
5. Hodgkin's disease

1. False
The granuloma of actinomycosis contain pus cells and the adherent filaments of the organism, the latter being known as the sulphur granules. Although the wall of an actinomycotic abscess is heavily infiltrated with lipid-laden macrophages no giant cells form.

2. False
The granulomas associated with schistosomiasis form around the eggs which are laid by the female in the veins of the walls of the lower urinary tract in the case of *S. haematobium*. Occasional epithelioid cells, fibroblasts, lymphocytes and plasma cells are seen but giant cells are not a special feature.

3. True
Primary biliary cirrhosis, a disease affecting women rather than men, is of unknown aetiology. Pathologically a non-suppurative process affects the intrahepatic bile ducts. Miliary granuloma form in the portal areas associated with a heavy infiltration of lymphoid cells and some giant cells.

4. False
In contradistinction to tuberculoid leprosy in which the lesions resemble those of tuberculosis giant cells are rarely found in the lepromatous variety of this

disease. In lepromatous leprosy the lesions consist of aggregates of macrophages which contain huge numbers of lepra bacilli. The bacilli tend not to be destroyed and to multiply within the cells which have ingested them.

5. True
The characteristic cell of Hodgkin's disease is the Sternberg–Reed giant cell. This cell possesses double mirror image nuclei and is a particular feature of the pleomorphic cellular infiltrate which replaces the normal lymphoid tissue. The cells are probably neoplastic cells derived from the mononuclear phagocyte system.

3.7 The following predispose to the development of tuberculosis:

1. HLA–B27
2. Sarcoidosis
3. Silicosis
4. Avitaminosis D
5. Malnutrition

1. False
The histocompatibility antigen HLA–B27 is not associated with an increased predisposition to tuberculosis but is associated with a high incidence of ankylosing spondylitis and acute anterior uveitis.

2. False
Tuberculosis is rarely associated with sarcoidosis and the tuberculin reaction is frequently negative. However, the pathological lesion in the lungs and lymph nodes resembles that of a tuberculoid granuloma but without any associated caseation.

3. True
There appears to be a synergism between silica and tuberculosis and in the presence of the former the incidence of the latter is greatly increased. When the mycobacterium becomes established the disease may rapidly progress terminating in tuberculous bronchopneumonia and miliary tuberculosis.

4. False
Although vitamin D was used in the treatment of tuberculosis and particularly for lupus vulgaris, there

is no evidence that a deficiency of this vitamin predisposes to the development of tuberculosis any more than a general state of malnutrition.

5. True
Protein-calorie malnutrition results in low resistance to a wide range of infections. Children with kwashiorkor have a depressed tuberculin reactivity and a lowered resistance to infection with mycobacteria.

3.8 Direct evidence of immunological activity can be demonstrated in the following chronic inflammatory diseases:

1. Lepromatous leprosy
2. Tuberculoid leprosy
3. Silicosis
4. Rheumatoid arthritis
5. Asbestosis

1. False
The granuloma associated with lepromatous leprosy consists of diffuse collections of foamy macrophages packed with globi of mycobacteria. No significant infiltration of lymphocytes or plasma cells occurs around these lesions and the lepromin test is negative.

2. True
Tuberculoid leprosy causes a non-caseating epithelioid cell granuloma in which the typical lesion is surrounded by a dense cuff of lymphocytes. The lepromin test is positive and evidence of T-lymphocyte activation can be found *in vitro*.

3. False
Patients suffering from silicosis may develop auto-antibodies but these are not directly involved in the pathogenesis of the silicotic nodules which are formed from collagen. Colloidal silica is intensely toxic to macrophages and it is this damage, with the release of intracellular lysosomes, which appears to stimulate the intense fibroblastic activity.

4. True
The microscopic appearance of the early lesions in rheumatoid arthritis is evidence of the immunological aetiology of this disease. Such lesions consist of a

111

central area of necrosis and fibroblastic activity surrounded by a cuff of lymphocytes and plasma cells.
The latter appear to produce the rheumatoid factor
which is an IgM anti-immunoglobulin antibody.

5. False
No evidence of immunological activity is seen in the
lesions produced by asbestos, another silica containing material which in fibre form can react with the
macrophage cell membrane to cause intense fibroblastic activity and collagen synthesis. When inhaled
this reactive lesion is found particularly around the
terminal bronchioles as well as the air sacs.

**3.9 Epithelioid cell granuloma formation is associ-
ated with the following diseases:**

1. Ulcerative colitis
2. Crohn's disease
3. Chronic glomerulo-nephritis
4. Toxoplasmosis
5. Sarcoidosis

1. False
This condition, which is a chronic inflammatory
disease of the colon, is not associated with granuloma formation. Characteristically the disease, in its
later and more severe forms, is associated with
mucosal denudation due to the coalescence of
smaller ulcers which develop from crypt abscesses.
Such ulceration seldom extends more deeply than
the submucosa.

2. True
The lesions of Crohn's disease are typical epithelioid
cell granulomas. These occur in 60 per cent of all
cases and may extend through the muscle of the
intestine to involve the peritoneal surface of the gut.
Fibrosis becomes increasingly prominent in more
chronic cases.

3. False
Organised granulomas do not occur in this condition
although fibrosis develops around the glomerular
tuft leading to its deformation. This disease is attributed to chronic immune complex deposition.

4. True

Small epithelioid cell granulomas may be a feature of the lesions of toxoplasmosis, a disease caused by the protozoon, *Toxoplasma gondii*. They may be found in the enlarged lymph nodes which typically occur in this infection.

5. True

Sarcoidosis is a disease of unknown aetiology in which the lesions found in the lungs and lymph nodes are typically non-caseating tuberculoid granulomas. These may be followed by intense pulmonary fibrosis. The intradermal injection of an extract of spleen from another individual with sarcoidosis will produce an organised epithelioid cell granuloma maximal 6 weeks after injection (Kveim test) in affected individuals.

3.10 Organised epithelioid cell granulomas develop in the following infections:

1. Leprosy
2. Syphilis
3. Ankylostomiasis
4. Ascariasis
5. Schistosomiasis

1. True

Epithelioid granulomas develop in the tuberculoid and not in the lepromatous form of leprosy. In the former the granulomas are immunologically induced and the positive Mitsuda type of skin reaction which develops within 2 to 3 weeks of the intradermal injection of dead *Mycobacterium leprae* is also an epithelioid cell granuloma. In contrast the granulomas associated with lepromatous leprosy are not immunologically induced, contain no epithelioid cells and the Mitsuda test is negative.

2. True

The gummas formed in tertiary syphilis have the appearance of immunologically induced granulomas. They are surrounded by an extensive zone of lymphocytes and plasma cells. Epithelioid cells may be found in follicles together with giant cells, the latter being smaller than the Langhan's cells found in tuberculosis.

3. False

Hookworm infection is not associated with granuloma formation. Transient pulmonary eosinophilia occurs in this condition if the larvae penetrate the intestinal wall and migrate through the lungs. Individuals suffering from ankylostomiasis usually have a severe anaemia due to the induced gastrointestinal haemorrhage.

4. False

Ascariasis is not associated with granuloma formation. This intestinal infestation caused by the round worm, *Ascaris lumbricoides*, is particularly prevalent in tropical areas. Migration of the larvae causes pulmonary eosinophilia and individuals harbouring the worm commonly have a circulating eosinophilia and high IgE levels. A common complication, however, is cholangitis due to the worms migrating into and obstructing the common bile duct.

5. True

The granulomas formed round schistosome eggs in the liver, intestines and bladder are typical immunologically induced epithelioid cell granulomas, usually associated with lymphocytes, plasma cells and eosinophils. Large numbers of fibroblasts are present and so these lesions are followed by intense fibrosis.

3.11 The following metals cause epithelioid cell granulomas:

1. Beryllium
2. Chromium
3. Zirconium
4. Nickel
5. Iron

1. True

The inhalation of beryllium is followed by a chronic inflammatory response in the lung. Fibrosis follows and commonly a non-caseating tuberculoid reaction is seen in the tissues. In addition to this action beryllium is a contact sensitising metal.

2. False

Potassium dichromate does not cause granuloma

114

formation but it does cause severe contact sensitivity. This particularly affects workers in the building trade because it may be a constituent of cement. Chromium used in orthopaedic implants can also cause sensitisation leading to local tissue breakdown, as well as generalised skin rashes.

3. True
The metal itself is inert. However, zirconium lactate can cause non-caseating tuberculoid granulomas in the skin, the development of which are due to delayed hypersensitivity.

4. False
Nickel does not cause granulomas but like potassium dichromate it is a contact sensitiser. It may also give rise to local tissue reactions if used in orthopaedic implants.

5. False
No tissue reaction occurs in response to iron or its various salts. However, in persons who have inhaled iron compounds over long periods an X-ray of the lungs gives a false impression that multiple granulomas have developed. No evidence of a chronic inflammatory lesion is, however, found in lung biopsies performed in such individuals.

Section 4. HOSPITAL AND WOUND INFECTION

4.1. Infection within a hospital may be:

1. dust-borne
2. water-borne
3. food-borne
4. hand-borne
5. endogenous

1. True
The spread of respiratory tract infections may occur by the inhalation of infected particles in the air. These may have been redistributed by the dusting of furniture or bed making.

2. True
Water-borne infection may occur due to contamina-

tion of a water supply with excreta. This is the common method of spread of cholera and typhoid fever.

3. True
Food-borne infection is usually the result of infection of the food supplied to patients by foodhandlers who are carrying an intestinal pathogen. Alternatively if infected water is used for washing food infection may be transmitted.

4. True
Hand-borne infections are usually due to poor personal hygiene. Patients and carriers with intestinal pathogens can contaminate their hands with traces of faeces when cleansing themselves after defaecation.

5. True
Endogenous infection is common particularly in patients in whom the original disease was the result of bacterial infection, e.g. peritonitis following appendicitis or diverticulitis.

4.2 General factors predisposing to wound infection include:

1. uncontrolled diabetes
2. hypogammaglobulinaemia
3. low platelet count
4. agranulocytopenia
5. eosinophilia

1. True
The defective carbohydrate metabolism of diabetes results in a diminished supply of energy for the polymorphonuclear leucocytes, thus diminishing their phagocytic potential.

2. True
Because all antibodies are gammaglobulins it follows that hypogammaglobulinaemia is associated with a failure of antibody formation and hence the reduction of one of the important factors concerned in resistance to infection.

3. True
This statement is true because severe thrombocy-

116

topenia predisposes to the development of a wound haematoma, a common precursor of wound infection.

4. True
Since polymorphonuclear leucocytes are a major factor in controlling infection by pathogenic microorganisms if these cells are absent an increased susceptibility to infection results and any infection which does occur tends to be more dangerous.

5. False
The eosinophil leucocyte is concerned with parasitic infestation by various kinds of worm rather than with pyogenic infections.

4.3 The following diseases are the result of arthropod-borne blood infections:

1. Cholera
2. Trypanosomiasis
3. Tetanus
4. Malaria
5. Hydatid disease

1. False
Cholera is a water-borne infection, transmission taking place by the faecal-oral route.

2. True
Trypanosomiasis is transmitted by the tsetse fly. *T. gambiense* is transmitted mainly by intra-human cycles whereas *T. rhodesiense* is a zoonosis.

3. False
Tetanus is due to the Gram-positive *Clostridium tetani* which is found in the soil often in spore form. Following injury the spore contaminates the wound and develops into the vegetative toxin producing form only if conditions are anaerobic.

4. True
Malaria is transmitted by the anopheles mosquito. The disease is caused by one of four species of plasmodium: *Plasmodium vivax, malariae, ovale* or *falciparum*. The latter is the most important.

5. False

Hydatid disease is caused by the tapeworms, *Echinococcus granulosus* and *multilocularis*. The natural cycle is from dog to sheep and man is infected only by accident.

4.4 *Streptococcus faecalis*:

1. is a common inhabitant of the gastrointestinal tract
2. grows in long chains
3. flourishes in bile-salt lactose media
4. is concerned in the aetiology of periodontal disease
5. is an opportunistic rather than a true pathogen

1. True

Streptococcus faecalis is almost as numerous in the faeces of man as the bacteroides, bifidobacteria and enterobacteriaceae.

2. False

This organism occurs in pairs looking like spectacles or at the most, in short chains.

3. True

Streptococcus faecalis grows on MacConkey's medium and other bile-salt lactose media to produce very small pink colonies. Normally no change occurs on a blood agar plate although a variant exists which causes a clear zone of haemolysis without producing a soluble haemolysin.

4. True

The superficial dental plaques which form in the angle around the crown of the tooth just above the margin of the gum are inhabited by *Streptococcus mutans*, *mitis* and *faecalis*. When the mouth is not kept clean this marginal plaque grows down into the gingival crevice and induces a change in the bacterial flora to one dominated by anaerobic Gram negative cocci, bacilli, vibrios and spirochaetes. The toxins and enzymes produced by these various organisms accompanied by the immune response to their antigens damages the periodontal tissues causing the development of gingivitis and pyorrhoea.

5. True
Streptococcus faecalis is an opportunistic pathogen. Unlike a true pathogen it can only produce a pathological lesion in the presence of a lowered tissue resistance or abnormal environmental conditions.

4.5 The virulence of bacteria is related to:

1. their number in the tissues
2. the production of toxins
3. their ability to produce spreading factors
4. their resistance to phagocytosis
5. decreased resistance of the host

1. False
The number of bacteria does not affect their virulence, only their potential for producing an infective lesion. About 10^5 coagulase positive staphylococci are required to produce a superficial infective lesion such as a boil.

2. True
Bacterial toxins are of two main types, exotoxins and endotoxins. Both play a large part in determining bacterial virulence. The former, which are mainly produced by Gram-positive organisms, diffuse freely from the organisms into the surrounding tissues although some, like the exotoxin of *Clostridium tetani* have an affinity for specific tissues. Endotoxins, however, are an integral part of the cell. Typical examples are the glyco-lipid complexes of the Gram-negative organisms such as *Escherichia coli*.

3. True
Spreading factors such as streptokinase, which are produced by *Streptococcus pyogenes*, are important factors in determining bacterial virulence. This enzyme activates a proteolytic enzyme precursor in the plasma and causes the lysis of fibrin clots. Another factor of similar importance is hyaluronidase which is produced by *Clostridium perfringens* and other organisms. This enzyme splits hyaluronic acid, the muco-polysaccharide intercellular cement substance, enabling the clostridia to spread along the tissue planes.

119

4. True

Resistance to phagocytosis chiefly depends upon the presence of surface components on the bacteria which make it difficult for the phagocytic cells to ingest them. Virulent strains of pneumococci, for example, possess polysaccharide capsules. Rough mutants of pneumococci which have lost their capsules are readily engulfed by phagocytes.

5. False

Decreased resistance of the host does not affect the inherent virulence of the organism. It does, however, affect the number required to produce a clinical lesion. In an experimental animal the minimum lethal dose of organisms would also be reduced.

4.6 Bacteria are normally found on or in the:

1. blood
2. urinary tract
3. lower bronchi
4. gastrointestinal tract
5. skin, sebaceous glands and hair follicles

1. False

In a normal individual bacteria are only transiently found in the blood stream, e.g. following tooth brushing. Such bacteria do not multiply and are rapidly eliminated.

2. False

The urinary tract is normally sterile. Infection of the female urethra with Gram negative cocci, however, is the common cause of the urethral syndrome, often mistakenly referred to as 'cystitis' although the bladder urine is sterile.

3. False

The lower bronchi are normally sterile.

4. True

The gastrointestinal tract is inhabited by an abundant bacterial flora from the level of the duodeno-jejunal junction downwards. It has only recently been appreciated, however, that obligate anaerobes belonging to the bacteroides group constitute a majority of the intestinal flora. Prior to culture of the small bowel contents using anaerobic techniques it was thought that this part of the bowel was sterile.

5. True
Staphylococcus albus, *Staphylococcus aureus*, diphtheroid organisms, lactobacilli and a variety of obligate anaerobes colonise the skin and its appendages.

4.7 Pseudomembranous enterocolitis is caused by the following organisms:

1. *Clostridium sporogenes*
2. *Clostridium difficile*
3. *Streptococcus faecalis*
4. Penicillin resistant staphylococci
5. *Pseudomonas aeruginosa*

1. False
Clostridium sporogenes is one of the causative organisms of gas gangrene, it plays no part in the development of enterocolitis.

2. True
Clostridium difficile has recently been identified as the causal agent of antibiotic associated colitis. The organism is resistant to both lincomycin and clindamycin and exerts its noxious effect through the production of cytopathic toxin. The organism is sensitive to vancomycin and metranidazole.

3. False
Streptococcus faecalis plays no part in the development of pseudomembranous enterocolitis. This organism is an opportunistic pathogen and can only produce a pathological lesion when tissue resistance is lowered.

4. True
Penicillin resistant staphylococci are believed to play a part in the development of one type of pseudomembranous enterocolitis. This type was particularly common in the past when broad spectrum antibiotics were commonly used for prophylaxis against wound infection.

5. False
Pseudomonas aeruginosa plays no part in the development of pseudomembranous enterocolitis. This or-

ganism is of considerable importance, however, in burns when the burnt surface tends to be colonised by this organism producing the characteristic greenish pus.

4.8 The major pathogens in post operative chest infections are:

1. *Haemophilus influenzae*
2. *Streptococcus pyogenes*
3. *Mycobacterium tuberculosis*
4. *Staphylococcus aureus*
5. *Streptococcus pneumoniae*

1. True
This organism is one of the most important pathogens concerned in the development of post operative chest infections particularly in patients in whom pulmonary collapse occurs. This organism is sensitive to the antibiotic cefamandole.

2. False
This organism plays no part in the development of post operative pulmonary infection. It is, however, an important pathogen causing acute tonsillitis, impetigo, wound infections, otitis media, scarlet and rheumatic fever.

3. False
Mycobacterium tuberculosis, although a cause of severe chronic pulmonary infection, plays no part in the development of post operative chest infection.

4. True
Staphylococcus aureus may be of importance in post operative chest infections but only in the presence of a staphylococcal septicaemia. A typical lesion of multiple small abscesses develops within the lungs.

5. True
Streptococcus pneumoniae is the chief pathogenic invader of the lungs, normally producing lobar pneumonia. Since post operative pulmonary infection is normally limited to areas involved in collapse the classical picture does not develop. It should also be noted that the majority of pathogenic bacteria, chlamydia, rickettsia, viruses and fungi are potential

causes of post operative chest infection although all are uncommon.

4.9 The following bacteria are commonly found in infected wounds following colonic operations:

1. *Escherichia coli*
2. *Neisseria meningitidis*
3. *Streptococcus pyogenes*
4. *Streptococcus faecalis*
5. *Bacteroides fragilis*

1. True
Escherichia coli belongs to a group of bacteria known as the *Enterobacteriaceae*, many members of which are responsible for wound infections. Other than *E.coli* these include *Klebsiella aerogenes* and *Proteus mirabilis*.

2. False
Neisseria meningitidis is a coccal organism, normally a commensal in the nasopharynx which plays no part in wound infection but is, of course, the causal organism of acute meningococcal meningitis.

3. True
A microaerophilic streptococcus may be involved in wound infection following colonic operations. If combined with other organisms such as *Proteus mirabilis* or *Staphylococcus aureus* a progressive synergistic gangrene may develop often referred to as Melaney's synergistic gangréné. This type of gangrene is particularly common in obese patients, black necrotic sloughs developing on the abdominal wall.

4. True
Streptococcus faecalis is a commensal of the large intestine and may be involved in any wound infection following colonic surgery.

5. True
The part played by *Bacteroides fragilis* has only recently been appreciated since it was common clinical practice to culture all wound swabs taken from infected wounds under aerobic conditions. Since *Bact. fragilis* is a strict anaerobe its presence was, therefore, unrecognised.

4.10 The incidence of postoperative infection can be reduced by the use of the following measures:

1. The use of negative pressure ventilation in the operating theatre
2. The use of filtered air in the operating theatre, pore size 10 μm
3. Showering by the surgeon and all attendants prior to embarking upon the operation
4. The administration of prophylactic antibiotics
5. Disinfection of the patient's skin prior to operation

1. False
The most commonly used system of theatre ventilation is a positive pressure (plenum) system. Although there are various methods by which this can be achieved the downward displacement method is the most popular. In this type of system filtered air is introduced into the theatre from ports in the ceiling and air is extracted from floor level.

2. False
This is too large. The most commonly used filters have pores of approximately 5 μm in diameter. Pores smaller than this are unnecessary since the organisms are never solitary but are usually to be found on dust particles. One difficulty encountered with a smaller pore size is the difficulty of maintaining the filters which rapidly become blocked.

3. False
Showering is not a practice which is to be recommended since it removes the oil from the surface skin to which organisms normally adhere. The result is that any movement by the surgeon or attendants will be attended by a shower of organisms.

4. True
Prophylactic antibiotics have been shown to be effective in reducing the incidence of post operative wound infection in a variety of potentially infective conditions such as acute appendicitis and colonic operations. At the present time clindamycin or metronidazole are being used with increasing frequency.

5. True
Disinfection of the patient's skin prior to surgery

is regarded as an essential prerequisite of aseptic surgery. This may be carried out by a variety of materials. At present the iodophors or chlorhexidine are commonly used for this purpose.

4.11 Renal tract infection is caused by a variety of bacteria including:

1. *Streptococcus pyogenes*
2. *Klebsiella pneumoniae*
3. *Streptococcus faecalis*
4. *Staphylococcus aureus*
5. *Escherichia coli*

1. False
This organism is associated with the development of progressive glomerulonephritis. In this latter situation fluorescent microscopy reveals a granular deposition of IgG and complement in the walls of the glomerular capillaries.

2. True
Otherwise known as *Freidlander's bacillus* this organism is most commonly found in mixed infections and in the presence of structural deformities of the urinary tract.

3. True
This organism is a particularly common offender following catheterisation in women.

4. True
Both *Staphylococcus albus* (Coag−ve) and *Staphylococcus aureus* (Coag+ve) can cause pyelonephritis. The former more commonly than the latter. The Coagulase +ve organism is only occasionally found in structurally abnormal urinary tracts.

5. True
This organism is the commonest cause of acute and chronic urinary tract infection.

4.12 Staphylococci pathogenic to man:

1. produce a capsular polysaccharide
2. grow in irregular clusters in culture
3. produce coagulase

4. are resistant to penicillin
5. all produce an enterotoxin

1. False
Capsular polysaccharide is associated with the pathogenic forms of pneumococci. The presence of a capsule produces the smooth variant, loss of the capsule an avirulent rough form.

2. True
The growth of the staphylococci is irregular thus producing irregular clusters.

3. True
The ability to produce coagulase, an enzyme which clots citrated plasma *in vitro*, differentiates the pathogenic forms of staphylococci from the non-pathogenic.

4. False
Pathogenic staphylococci are not necessarily resistant to penicillin although most strains associated with epidemic and endemic disease in hospitals in fact are resistant. Resistance to this, or any other antibiotics, affects the treatment of an infection but not the initial pathogenicity of the organisms.

5. False
Only some strains of staphylococci produce an enterotoxin. Food containing such organisms acts as a culture medium and when ingested the toxin gives rise to giddiness, vomiting and diarrhoea. This is often severe but recovery usually occurs within a day or two.

4.13 The common pathogenic pyogenic organisms affecting man include:

1. *Staphylococcus aureus*
2. *Clostridium tetani*
3. *Staphylococcus albus*
4. Bacteroides
5. *Pseudomonas aeruginosa*

1. True
The pathogenic varieties of this Gram positive organism are particularly associated with:

126

(a) The development of localised infections such as boils, carbuncles and abscesses

(b) Spreading infections of the skin such as impetigo

(c) Septicaemia followed by the formation of pyogenic abscesses, osteomyelitis or endocarditis

2. False

Clostridium tetani is not a pyogenic organism. It causes its pathogenic effects by an exotoxin which diffuses up the peripheral or cranial motor nerves to reach the spinal cord or brain where it interferes with the normal inhibitory control of the lower motor neurones by the higher centres.

3. False

Staphylococcus albus is a commensal and rarely pathogenic; it is extremely common on the skin.

4. True

The bacteroides are the commonest bacteria inhabiting the gastrointestinal tract. They are a particularly important cause of pus formation in surgical wounds following colo-rectal surgery.

5. True

Normally present in small numbers in the gastrointestinal tract these organisms can cause severe infections in burn patients. The pus produced possesses a characteristic greenish colour. These organisms are also responsible for some urinary tract infections and may invade the blood stream to produce a septicaemia.

Section 5. DISINFECTION, STERILISATION AND ANTIBIOTICS

5.1 When using an autoclave to sterilise surgical drapes and instruments it is essential that:

1. the load should be tightly packed
2. the containers in which the loads are packed should be impervious to steam
3. air should be completely removed from the chamber prior to the admission of steam
4. a vacuum must be made at the end of the cycle

5. an adequate indication of autoclave efficiency should be included in the load

1. False
The loads should not be tightly packed because tight packing hinders the passage of steam into and through the loads thus interfering with sterilisation.

2. False
The containers must be porous to allow the admission of steam. If metal drums are used these should possess vents for the admission of steam and these vents should be checked before the drums are placed in the autoclave to make certain they are open.

3. True
This is a prerequisite for the correct functioning of the modern autoclave which does not depend on gravity displacement. By removing 98 per cent of the air from the chamber penetration of the load occurs almost instantly so that more efficient sterilisation is obtained and the cycle time is shortened.

4. True
The creation of a vacuum at the end of the cycle in a chamber still warm from the presence of steam, in both the chamber and the surrounding jacket, ensures that the contents of the autoclave are dry before removal.

5. True
Adequate indication of satisfactory sterilisation can be obtained by the use of autoclave tapes. These are frequently adhesive tapes on which are imprinted diagonal grey shaded lines which change into a dark colour after being exposed to the correct amount of heat, the Bowie–Dick test.

5.2 Spores are killed by exposure to:

1. moist heat at 110°C for 15 minutes
2. dry heat at 160°C for 1 hour
3. ethylene oxide
4. hydrogen peroxide
5. gentian violet

1. False
Bacterial spores require exposure to moist heat at a

temperature of 121°C for at least 15 minutes and preferably 30 minutes before they are destroyed. Resistant spores such as the spores of *Clostridium botulinum* can resist autoclaving at the lower temperature of 115°C for up to 40 minutes.

2. True
The majority of spores are killed by exposure to dry heat at 160°C for 1 hour. In practice this is an unacceptable method of sterilisation because slight charring of paper and cotton occurs at this temperature.

3. True
Ethylene oxide is highly lethal to all kinds of microbes and spores. It is of particular value for sterilising articles liable to damage by heat, e.g. plastic and rubber articles. Sterilisation time depends upon the temperature of the reaction and the relative humidity.

4. False
Hydrogen peroxide has been used as an antiseptic but has little or no action on bacterial spores.

5. False
Gentian violet will kill some vegetative forms of bacteria particularly Gram positive organisms, it is much less active against Gram negative bacteria and virtually useless against spores of any kind.

5.3 Differences between disinfectants and antiseptics are:

1. The latter are more harmful to living tissue cells
2. Antiseptics free inanimate objects from vegetative organisms whereas disinfectants are used for the local removal of pathogenic bacteria from the tissues
3. The former are more readily inactivated by contact with proteinaceous material such as blood
4. The speed of action of the former can be accelerated by raising the temperature whereas the action of the latter can only be increased by increasing their concentration
5. There are specific differences in the mode of action of both groups of compounds

1. False
The converse is correct.

2. False
The converse is correct. Disinfectants are used to free inanimate objects from vegetative organisms but not necessarily from spores whereas antiseptics are primarily bacteriostatic agents for the removal of pathogenic bacteria from the tissues.

3. False
Both are equally affected by proteinaceous material.

4. False
The speed of action of both groups of substances can be accelerated by raising the temperature and/or their concentration.

5. False
Both groups of agents may have a variety of actions including disruption of the cytoplasmic membranes, enzyme systems or cellular proteins.

5.4 Chemical agents used as disinfectants and antiseptics include the following compounds:

1. The phenols
2. Isopropyl alcohol
3. The halogens
4. The soaps
5. Derivatives of salicylic acid

1. True
Phenol, which is carbolic acid, was used by Lister over 100 years ago, to prevent wound infection. This group of chemical compounds act by coagulating protein. Phenol is effective against both bacteria and viruses but it is no longer used because of its toxicity. However, a variety of derivatives such as lysol, Dettol and hexachlorophine are in common use.

2. True
This compound is in common use for sterilisation of the skin, it is most effective in 70 per cent concentration. The alcohols act by coagulating cell proteins and will kill bacteria and some viruses.

3. True
The halogens, or any substance capable of releasing

them, such as sodium hypochlorite, are lethal to bacteria, viruses, fungi and spores. Their action is to oxidise SH groups but a disadvantage is their susceptibility to quenching by organic matter.

4. True
Soaps have weak disinfectant activity although they are active against *Strep. pyogenes*, *Strep. pneumoniae*, *Haemophilus influenzae* and the virus of influenza. They have no action on *Staph. pyogenes*, mycobacteria or Gram-negative bacilli. The main effect of soap is a mechanical one removing the transient skin flora.

5. False
Salicylic acid and the salicylates have no disinfectant or antiseptic action.

5.5 The following antibiotics are effective against fungi:

1. Nystatin
2. Bacitracin
3. Griseofulvin
4. Polymyxin B
5. Amphotericin B

1. True
Candida albicans, *Cryptococcus neoformans* and *Histoplasma capsulatum* and *dubosii* are sensitive to this drug. However, the drug is not absorbed and, therefore, has no systemic effect. Its chief clinical use is, therefore, limited to oropharyngeal and skin infections caused by *Candida albicans*.

2. False
Bacitracin is a polypeptide antibiotic which is active against many Gram positive bacteria and neisseria. It is now only used locally for skin infections.

3. True
This drug, which was originally derived from a penicillium mould, inhibits the growth of the epidermophyton causing athlete's foot, the trichophyton causing ring worm and the microsporum causing tinea. Administered orally griseofulvin is partially

absorbed and is incorporated into the keratin of skin, nails and hair.

4. False
The polymyxins are polypeptides which are derived from the soil organisms *B. polymyxa*. Five have been identified of which two are in commercial use, polymyxin B (polymyxin) and polymyxin E (coliston). These drugs are effective against both Gram-positive and -negative organisms, particularly *Pseudomonas aeruginosa* but they are inactive against proteus. They have no antifungal action.

5. True
This drug is the most effective agent for the treatment of systemic fungal infections. It is active against *Histoplasma capsulatum* and *dubosii*, *Cryptococcus neoformans*, *Coccidioides immitis*, *Blastomyces dermatitidis* and *Candida albicans*.

5.6 Benzyl penicillin is:

1. bacteriostatic
2. destroyed by the enzyme penicillinase
3. insoluble in water
4. damaging to the nucleus of the bacterial cell
5. active against some viruses

1. False
Benzyl penicillin is bactericidal. *In vitro* bacteria which have been exposed to this antibiotic die even when transferred to a drug-free medium. Compare this with bacteriostatic drugs such as the tetracyclines. Exposure to a bacteriostatic antibiotic causes the cessation of bacterial growth but division recommences if the organisms are transferred to an antibiotic free medium.

2. True
Penicillinase destroys penicillin by hydrolysis to inactive penicilloic acid and by opening the β-lactam ring.

3. False
Benzyl penicillin is extremely soluble in water.

4. False
Penicillin exerts its bactericidal effect by its action

on the bacterial cell wall. It prevents the synthesis of the mucopeptide of the cell wall which renders the sensitive organism vulnerable to osmotic pressure.

5. False
Penicillin and the semisynthetic derivatives have no action on the viruses.

5.7 Bacteria resistant to benzyl penicillin include:

1. penicillinase-producing organisms
2. the majority of Gram-negative bacteria
3. Gram-positive anaerobic spore forming organisms
4. the Bacteroides
5. *Streptococcus pneumoniae*

1. True
Penicillinase causes a split in the penicillin molecule at the peptide linkage. This destroys the capacity of penicillin to interfere with the synthesis of the bacterial cell wall.

2. True
The majority of Gram-negative bacteria are resistant to the action of benzyl penicillin because the amount of mucopeptide in their cell walls is considerably less than in the Gram-positive cocci. In addition the greater complexity of the cell wall of Gram-negative organisms hinders penicillin from reaching the site of mucopeptide synthesis. However, some strains of *Escherichia coli*, *Salmonella typhi* and *Shigella* are sensitive to this drug.

3. False
Both the rod-like spore forming organisms responsible for gas gangrene and tetanus, which are Gram-positive, are sensitive to benzyl penicillin.

4. True
The bacteroides are sensitive only to lincomycin, clindamycin and metranidazole.

5. False
Streptococcus pneumoniae causing lobar pneumonia and the other streptococci responsible for meningi-

tis, otitis media and sinusitis are extremely sensitive to benzyl penicillin.

5.8 Antibiotics which inhibit the synthesis of mucopeptide in the wall of a bacterium include:

1. cycloserine
2. cephalosporins
3. neomycin
4. penicillin and its semisynthetic derivatives
5. erythromycin

1. True
D-cycloserine is a structural analogue of D-alanine and, therefore, effectively inhibits the formation of the dipeptide D-alanyl-D-alanine from D-alanine. This reaction is essential for mucopeptide synthesis and, therefore, the formation of the bacterial cell wall.

2. True
The cephalosporins inhibit the end stages of the synthesis of mucopeptide.

3. False
Neomycin is a bactericidal agent which acts by inhibiting protein synthesis. This antibiotic becomes bound to that part of the ribosomes which absorb transfer-RNA. One theory put forward to explain the action of this and other similar antibiotics such as streptomycin and kanamycin suggests that any messenger RNA molecules which reach ribosomes to which neomycin has become attached are 'misread' in the course of protein synthesis.

4. True
All penicillins act on the end stages of mucopeptide synthesis.

5. False
Erythromycin, a member of the macrolide group of antibiotics which includes sporamycin and oleandomycin, inhibits protein synthesis by mechanisms as yet unknown.

5.9 Ototoxicity is a well recognised complication following the administration of:

1. Streptomycin

2. Gentamicin
3. Neomycin
4. Bacitracin
5. Erythromycin

1. True
This is the most serious toxic effect of streptomycin. This antibiotic usually causes vestibular disturbance producing vertigo although true deafness occasionally occurs.

2. True
Gentamicin produces labyrinthine damage but this rarely occurs unless renal failure is present. This drug is excreted by the kidney and in the presence of renal failure high serum levels develop even after normal dose schedules, i.e. 80 mg thrice daily.

3. True
Neomycin can cause irreversible deafness and is the principal reason why this antibiotic is no longer used for systemic treatment.

4. False
This drug is nephrotoxic, not ototoxic. It is not used systemically.

5. False
Erythromycin is exceptionally safe. Erythromycin estolate is hepatotoxic but no other preparations possess this undesirable side effect.

Section 6. WOUND HEALING

6.1 Wound healing is enhanced by the administration of:

1. cortisol
2. zinc
3. aldosterone
4. oxygen
5. vitamin C

1. False
Cortisol impairs the synthesis of collagen and enhances its lysis and thus inhibits wound healing.

2. True
Zinc has been shown to accelerate the development of granulation tissue in a wound produced by the excision of a pilonidal sinus. The exact mechanism is unknown but there is evidence that it stabilises macromolecules and stimulates the biosynthesis of collagen.

3. False
Aldosterone has no effect in wound healing.

4. True
The fibroblast requires an ambient pO_2 of around 10 mm Hg in order to synthesise collagen and ground substance.

5. True
Although the administration of vitamin C does not accelerate wound healing a deficiency causes a reduction in the synthesis of collagen and hence a lack of proper healing. If the deficiency of vitamin C is severe and prolonged so that scurvy develops even wounds which have previously healed will break down.

6.2 Primary union of a wound is associated with the following:

1. a lag phase
2. a demolition phase
3. a contractile phase
4. a proliferative phase
5. a maturation phase

1. True
The lag phase is the first phase after suture of the wound. Little cellular activity occurs during this period and the integrity of the wound is preserved by the sutures.

2. True
This phase, of minimal duration in a clean incised wound, is associated with a mild inflammatory reaction at the wound edges. A little exudate occurs accompanied by the migration of polymorphonuclear leucocytes and later monocytes and lymphocytes.

3. False
Contraction is an essential feature of an open wound which is healing by secondary union (intention). Precisely how contraction occurs remains unknown although it may be caused by the fibroblasts of the granulation tissue, the myofibroblasts. The magnitude of contraction is greatest in sites where the skin is only loosely attached to the underlying tissues.

4. True
The proliferative phase begins as the demolition phase ends. Great activity of the fibroblast-capillary system occurs which forms a thin layer of granulation tissue between the two edges of the wound.

5. True
This is the terminal phase of wound healing. During maturation the tensile strength of the wound is gradually increased by intermolecular bonding between the collagen fibrils. In addition the collagen is remodelled in response to mechanical stress placed on the wound.

6.3 The healing of a wound is delayed by:

1. vitamin C deficiency
2. starvation
3. the administration of glucocorticoids
4. lack of blood supply
5. infection

1. True
Wound healing is dependent upon the synthesis of adequate amounts of collagen. This, in turn, is dependent upon the presence of vitamin C. Since man, monkey and the guinea-pig are unable to synthesise this vitamin its absence from the diet disturbs wound healing.

2. True
Starvation will affect wound healing but only when vitamin C deficiency has developed. Otherwise, even in markedly debilitated individuals, normal wound healing takes place.

3. True
The administration of excessive quantities of glucocorticoids causes a defect in collagen synthesis and in addition diminishes blood vessel formation.

4. True

A deficient blood supply leads to a lack of oxygen in the wound. This in turn diminishes fibroblastic activity because fibroblasts require an ambient O_2 tension of about 10 mm Hg in order to function correctly.

5. True

Infection retards collagen synthesis and enhances the breakdown of pre-existing collagen and hence delays wound healing.

6.4 Collagen, the ultimate source of the strength of a wound:

1. is formed by undifferentiated mesenchymal cells
2. is changed with the passage of time
3. undergoes lysis as well as synthesis even when the total collagen content of the wound is remaining constant
4. is broken down by the enzyme collagenase
5. is normally embedded in ground substance

1. False

Collagen is formed in the endoplasmic reticulum of the fibroblasts and excreted into the extracellular space in a monomeric form known as tropocollagen. When its synthesis is disturbed, as for example, in vitamin C deficiency, the precursor material collects and distorts the cell.

2. True

The protocollagen, which is the precursor material excreted into the extracellular space, is hydroxylated under the influence of the enzyme protocollagen hydroxylase. Polymerisation of the tropocollagen also occurs, strong covalent linkages being formed with neighbouring molecules.

3. True

The total amount of collagen in a wound may reach normal levels within 60 to 80 days but qualitative changes occur over a much longer period even though the total amount of collagen in the wound remains practically constant. Lysis is not confined to the wound but extends outwards from it for a variable distance. Should lysis be less intense than synthesis a hypertrophic or keloid scar may develop.

4. True
Collagenase is a naturally produced enzyme which is responsible for the breakdown of collagen. It has been shown in colonic anastomoses that up to 40 per cent of the old collagen is lost in the first 4 to 6 days. This loss of collagen is believed to be responsible for many cases of anastomotic breakdown.

5. True
The collagen fibres are embedded in a ground substance, the chemistry of which is as yet incompletely understood. A major component appears to be large protein-polysaccharide complexes called proteoglycans. Ground substance appears to play a role in the organised precipitation of collagen.

6.5 Post operative infection delays wound healing because:

1. the wound becomes packed with leucocytes
2. many of the organisms involved produce spreading factors which may destroy the intercellular ground substance
3. collagen is destroyed
4. capillary loops fail to develop
5. fibroblasts are diminished in number

1. False
Although the majority of infected wounds become infiltrated with leucocytes these do not delay wound healing. However, if the supply of oxygen is deficient phagocytic function is impaired and their capacity to kill ingested bacteria is diminished.

2. False
Spreading factors do not play a significant role in the delay of wound healing. They are, however, of great importance in the spread of a number of infections particularly gas gangrene.

3. True
Not only does infection lead to the destruction of pre-existing collagen it also retards collagen synthesis. Even in a normal incised wound collagenolysis

occurs for a distance of at least 5 mm on either side and is prominent for about one week.

4. False
Capillary loops, essential for the proper function of the fibroblasts, continue to develop in the presence of infection.

5. False
Fibroblasts continue to be produced but the formation of collagen is retarded and collagen which is formed undergoes collagenolysis.

6.6 The following are the features associated with the healing of open wounds:

1. The formation of granulation tissue
2. Infection
3. Migration of the surrounding epithelium
4. Giant cell formation
5. Contraction

1. True
Granulation tissue forms during the healing of both clean incised and open wounds, the difference is one of mass, less being formed during the healing of the former than the latter.

2. True
Some degree of infection is nearly always present when an open wound is present. In some circumstances this may be of great significance, e.g. infection of a burn wound by the haemolytic streptococcus may lead to a spreading infection and the destruction of any skin grafts which may be applied.

3. True
Migration of epithelial cells from the surrounding intact epithelium together with their proliferation leads to the formation of a sheet of cells which advances in a series of tongue-like projections beneath any remaining blood clot or exudate on the raw surface of the wound.

4. False
Giant cell formation will not be seen unless foreign material has been buried in the wound. This may then lead to the formation of foreign body giant cells.

5. True

Contraction is an important aspect of the healing of an open wound and it is most conspicuous when the skin is loose. It occurs to a remarkable extent in animals such as the rabbit. The mechanism bringing about contraction is still debatable but it probably arises from the contraction of the fibroblasts which, in addition to producing collagen, contain a contractile protoplasm similar to that found in muscle cells.

6.7 Wound healing may be governed by the following:

1. Trephones
2. Vitamin D
3. Chalones
4. Mineralocorticoids
5. The availability of sulphur containing aminoacids

1. True

It has been suggested that the stimulus to wound healing is mediated by trephones liberated by damaged cells. Although a working hypothesis based on tissue culture studies, the existence of such substances has yet to be proven *in vivo*.

2. False

Vitamin D is of little importance in the healing of soft tissue wounds.

3. True

This is a second hypothesis. It has been postulated that normal tissues secrete a substance capable of depressing mitosis, a chalone, and that a wound by removing some of this depressor substance permits an increased level of mitotic activity. There is some *in vitro* experimental work in the rabbit supporting this hypothesis although no chemical substance acting in this manner has yet been identified.

4. False

Mineralocorticoids play no specific part in wound healing but are, of course, of great importance in maintaining the optimal 'milieu interieux' without which normal body functions could not continue.

5. True

The presence of adequate amounts of sulphur containing amino acids such as methionine is essential for collagen synthesis. In well nourished individuals supplementing the diet with extra protein or additional vitamins, especially vitamin C, does not increase the rate of wound healing. The effects of protein and vitamin deficiency only become apparent in the starving animal.

6.8 Woven bone is found:

1. in bone forming in a model of cartilage
2. in fracture haematomas
3. in bones forming in sheets of differentiating mesenchyme
4. replacing lamellar bone in healing fractures
5. surrounding the ends of ununited fractures

1. False
Bone formed in a previous model of cartilage is of a lamellar type. Most of the skeleton is made of lamellar bone which replaces the initial cartilage, hence the term endochondral ossification. Lamellar bone is characterised by the arrangement of the collagen bundles into parallel sheets either forming concentric Haversian systems or flat plates.

2. True
Woven bone with its irregular arrangement of collagen bundles and osteocytes is the first type of bone forming in a fracture haematoma. It is replaced later by mature, lamellar or adult bone which is finally remodelled as the fracture unites.

3. True
Bone formed in differentiating mesenchyme is of the woven variety. This occurs during the embryonic development of the bones of the vault of the skull, the mandible and the clavicle. These bones being referred to as membrane bones.

4. False
The converse is true. Woven bone precedes lamellar bone.

5. False
The ends of ununited fractures are eventually covered by cartilage and if the latter are surrounded by

synovial cells a false joint or pseudarthrosis develops. At this stage union becomes impossible regardless of the duration of immobilisation.

6.9 The healing of a closed fracture may be associated with the following pathological consequences:

1. Myositis ossificans
2. Pseudarthrosis
3. Osteomyelitis
4. Osteosarcoma
5. Renal calculi

1. True
Immediately following injury a fracture haematoma forms, if the periosteum is torn, blood extends out into the surrounding tissues. Subsequent organisation and ossification leads to the development of myositis ossificans. This complication is particularly seen following fractures around the elbow joint and the pelvis.

2. True
The mesenchymal cells of the granulation tissue invading the fracture haematoma normally differentiate into bone forming osteoblasts which lay down woven bone. This is later replaced by lamellar bone. If, however, a fracture is imperfectly immobilised these cells may form fibrous tissue, cartilage and finally synovial cells with the result that a false joint develops. This is a well recognised complication of tibial fractures.

3. False
Infection of the fracture site is an extremely rare complication of an uncomplicated closed fracture. It might occasionally occur in patients suffering from multiple injuries in which a septicaemia develops due to infection elsewhere in the body.

4. False
Although the external callus around the fracture site may lead to a considerable 'tumour' there is no evidence that fractures lead to an increased incidence of osteosarcoma.

5. True
Fractures involving long term immobilisation parti-

cularly in the recumbent position may lead to renal calculi. These are often known as recumbency calculi and are due to the hypercalciuria which develops in an immobilised patient together with the relative stagnation of urine in the lowermost calyces of the kidney. Such calculi were, of course, much commoner in chronic spinal diseases, e.g. tuberculosis, prior to the development of the antituberculous drugs.

6.10 Ischaemic necrosis is a recognised complication of fractures of the following bones:

1. Talus
2. Calcaneum
3. Scaphoid
4. Pisiform
5. Femoral head

The answer is: 1, 3, 5 are **true** and 2 and 4 are **false**.

Ischaemic necrosis following fractures of the talus, scaphoid and femoral head is merely a reflection of the local peculiarities of the blood supply to these bones. Fracture lines running through these bones divorce one fragment from its blood supply with the result that ischaemic necrosis occurs. In fractures such as the femoral head the development of ischaemic necrosis will lead to pain once weight bearing begins. Radiologically the affected part becomes denser than the surrounding normal bone.

Section 7. IMMUNOLOGY

7.1 The following substances normally act as antigens, i.e. stimulate antibody production, when administered to humans:

1. Dextrans with a molecular weight below 150 000
2. Bovine insulin
3. Extracts of Primula
4. Human thyroglobulin
5. Rh.D. antigen

1. False
Dextrans with a molecular weight of less than 150 000

144

daltons can be used as plasma expanders without risk of antibody production. Carbohydrate above this weight are antigenic and carbohydrates below this weight become antigenic if conjugated with a protein.

2. True
Proteins exceeding a molecular weight of 10 000 are generally antigenic and although the molecular weight of bovine insulin is only 6000 this material evokes antibody production.

3. False
Extracts of the Primula have a molecular weight of only 210. They act, however, as haptens binding to the body's own protein through covalent linkages causing them to behave as antigens. This is a common cause of contact sensitivity in gardeners.

4. False
Normally the body does not react against its own thyroglobulin. However, in Hashimoto's thyroiditis autoimmune antibodies make their appearance in the circulation which are directed against thyroglobulin.

5. True
Immunisation with rhesus antigens occurs in:
 (a) Rh negative individuals transfused with Rh +ve blood
 (b) In some Rh −ve mothers following a pregnancy in which the foetus is Rh +ve

7.2 The following statements are true or false:

1. IgA is produced at mucous surfaces
2. IgM has a molecular weight of 150 000
3. IgE is the anaphylactic antibody
4. Antibody specificity depends on the constant regions of the F(ab) fragment
5. Immunoglobulin synthesis is dependent on thymic integrity in neonatal life

1. True
IgA is a very important immunoglobulin frequently secreted as a dimer (SIgA) conjugated to an epithelial glycoprotein of M.W. 50 000 referred to as the secre-

tory piece. The concentration of IgA in the saliva is 100 times that of IgG.

2. False
IgG has a molecular weight of 150 000. IgM consists of five such units together with additional carbohydrate. It has a molecular weight of 900 000 and the 'M' refers to macroglobulin. Blood group isoantibodies are IgM as are antibodies against *S. typhi* somatic antigens. Antibodies of the IgM class are frequently the first to be produced in an immune response.

3. True
IgE is the antibody involved in all anaphylactic reactions, binding to the surface of most cells. A reaction between IgE and an antigen results in the release of histamine, SRS-A (slow reacting substance of anaphylaxis), ECF-A (eosinophil chemotactic factor of anaphylaxis) and kallikrein. The latter is the enzyme that splits plasma kininogen to form kinins.

4. False
Antibody specificity towards antigen depends on the variable sequence of aminoacids in the adjoining heavy and light chains of the F(ab) fragment of the immunoglobulin molecule.

5. False
Immunoglobulins are secreted by plasma cells of the B-lymphocyte line, cells which are not under thymic control. In the chicken B-lymphocytes are under the control of the Bursa of Fabricius, hence their name. An equivalent organ has not, however, been identified in mammals. Mice thymectomised in neonatal life and children born with different types of thymic atresia do not possess T-lymphocytes but are still capable of producing immunoglobulins upon which humoral antibody responses depend.

7.3 Bence–Jones proteins are:

1. the heavy chains of immunoglobulins
2. found in the urine in multiple myeloma
3. associated with a monoclonal gammopathy
4. found in the urine in Waldenström's macroglobulinaemia
5. precipitated by boiling

1. False

Bence–Jones proteins are light chains not associated with the heavy chains which form normal immunoglobulins. They are secreted by the abnormal plasma cells in the condition known as multiple myeloma and pass from the plasma into the urine.

2. True

Bence–Jones proteins are only found in the urine in multiple myeloma. They are a necessary finding for the diagnosis of this disease. Additional diagnostic features of the disease are the presence of osteolytic deposits in the bones and abnormal plasma cells found on sternal marrow biopsy.

3. True

A monoclonal gammopathy together with the presence of an 'M' protein is a necessary feature of multiple myeloma but both are found in other conditions such as old age or following a massive immune response. In the latter conditions they are not associated with Bence–Jones proteins.

4. False

Multiple myeloma with Bence–Jones proteins is only associated with IgG, IgA, IgD or IgE, monoclonal gammopathies.

The corresponding condition for IgM is Waldenström's macroglobulinaemia in which the macroglobulin is not excreted in the urine. This syndrome is not associated with Bence–Jones proteins or osteolytic bony deposits but is found in men more often than women, especially over the age of fifty. The clinical features include weakness, spontaneous haemorrhage from mucosal surfaces, a susceptibility to infection and a variable degree of enlargement of the liver, spleen and lymph nodes.

5. False

Bence–Jones proteins precipitate at 80°C but return into solution on boiling. Other proteins in the urine are precipitated by boiling.

7.4 T-lymphocytes:

1. are immunoglobulin secreting cells
2. are found in the paracortical area of lymph nodes
3. are involved in contact dermatitis

4. are not involved in protection against tuberculosis
5. secrete lymphokines

1. False
T-lymphocytes do not produce or secrete immuno-globulins. They carry antibody-like receptor groups on their surface which specifically react with antigen. These are related to antigen reactive sites on the immunoglobulins as they have the same idiotypes. Anti-idiotypic antibodies produced against immunoglobulin idiotypes react with T-lymphocytes responding to the same antigen.

2. True
The paracortical areas of the lymph nodes lie between the true cortex and the corticomedullary junction which is the site of the post-capillary venules with their high walled endothelium. These areas become depleted of lymphocytes in neonatally thymectomised mice and in children born with thymic atresia and because of this the paracortical areas are sometimes known as the thymus dependent areas.

3. True
Contact dermatitis is the result of T-cell mediated immunity which is a reaction to antigen fixed in the periphery similar to skin allograft rejection. In man, contact dermatitis may be caused by simple metal haptens, such as nickel and potassium dichromate or by simple organic compounds such as dinitro-chlorobenzene, substances which bind to skin proteins through covalent linkages. Other contact agents include formalin, the epoxy resin hardeners used in the electronics industry and compounds used in rubber manufacture.

4. False
Mycobacteria such as *M. tuberculosis* and *M. leprae* are facultative intracellular parasites which tend to reside within macrophages. Host resistance to *M. tuberculosis* is produced by a reaction between specifically sensitised T-lymphocytes and mycobacterial antigen. These cells then secrete lymphokines which activate the macrophages causing increased activity of the hexose monophosphate shunt and the intracellular formation of bactericidal superoxides.

5. True

Both T and B-lymphocytes will, under certain circumstances, secrete lymphokines when activated by specific antigen or mitogens such as phytohaemagglutinins or concanavalin-A. The activity of this group of substances includes migration inhibitory factor (MIF), mitogenic factor, lymphotoxin, skin reactive factor (SRF) and macrophage activators. In addition both T and B-cells produce chemotactic factors and interferon.

7.5 The major histocompatibility complex (MHC) in man:

1. is situated in chromosome 6
2. has three loci controlling five groups of histocompatibility antigens
3. is involved in the expression of immune response (Ir) genes
4. shows a positive association with Hodgkin's disease, multiple sclerosis and ankylosing spondylitis
5. is tested for by the laboratory on a serum sample

1. True

The major histocompatibility complex consists of four loci situated on chromosome 6 in man. These control four groups of histocompatibility antigens HLA-A, B, C and D. The A and B group of antigens are serologically determined and the D locus antigens are mainly determined by mixed lymphocyte reaction.

2. False

Four loci control four groups of histocompatibility antigens (see 1). One antigen in each group is inherited from the father and one from the mother. HLA-D (related) antigens are found mainly on B-lymphocytes and these are coded for either by HLA-D or a very closely linked locus. Recently D related antigens have been discovered serologically and are referred to as HLA-DR.

3. True

HLA-D and HLA-DR are considered to be equivalent to the I region of the MHC in the mouse. (Ir) genes coded in this area which are autosomal dominant and inherited in a strictly Mendelian fashion are responsible for the immune response to a number of antigens.

4. True
Hodgkin's disease shows positive association with A1 and B8, multiple sclerosis with A3, B7 and DW2 and ankylosing spondylitis with B8.

5. False
HLA antigens are identified by the use of leucocyte suspensions. The term HLA is an abbreviation of the words human leucocyte antigens. Unclotted blood is needed by the laboratory.

7.6 Macrophages:

1. are not involved in the recognition of antigens
2. do not secrete lysosomal enzymes
3. can carry antibody on their surface
4. are involved in the tuberculin reaction
5. are important in graft rejection

1. False
Macrophages are important in antigen recognition, immune response genes being expressed by macrophages as well as lymphocytes. The macrophages process antigen which frequently results in the production of a more immunogenic material.

2. False
These cells secrete lysosomal and other enzymes such as hydrolases and proteases which are important factors in the processing of antigenic material in the phagosomes after phagocytosis. Such enzymes are also involved in degrading infecting microorganisms.

3. True
Macrophages have membrane receptors for the Fc fragment of some cytophilic antibodies which are then carried on the macrophage to their site of action.

4. True
Macrophages are a major feature of delayed hypersensitivity reactions. They form 50 per cent of the mononuclear cell infiltrate and are drawn to the site

of the reaction by lymphokines; macrophage chemotactic factors. The release of their lysosomal enzymes is probably a major factor in the development of the inflammatory reaction.

5. True
The cellular infiltrate accompanying the rejection of a skin graft is similar to that observed in a delayed hypersensitivity reaction. In both, the release of lysosomal hydrolytic enzymes from the macrophages is an important factor leading to tissue destruction.

7.7 Autoimmunity:

1. occurs because of a breakdown in the ability of the body to distinguish between self and non-self
2. is involved in some forms of orchitis
3. is involved in the production of cryoglobulins
4. is important in the pathogenesis of lupus erythematosus
5. does not result in immune complex disease

1. True
Substances of specific chemical structure and molecular weight behave as antigens if the body has not had contact with them before late fetal or early neonatal life. If such contact has been made then a substance is recognised as 'self' and no immunological reaction to its presence occurs. If, however, 'self' for some reason cannot be distinguished from 'non-self' a reaction known as the autoimmune response occurs with the production of antibodies known as 'autoantibodies'. Such a breakdown in the mechanisms associated with the recognition of potentially antigenic materials which are normally accepted by the body may follow an infection with viruses or mycoplasma, therapy with certain drugs or because a normal tissue barrier is broken down. The incidence of autoantibodies and the phenomena which they produce increases with age.

2. True
The orchitis seen in the human male associated with viral infections such as mumps may be due to an autoimmune type of reaction. Certainly an orchitis can be induced in animals by immunising them with testicular tissue in Freund's adjuvant.

3. True

Cryoglobulins are complexes of immunoglobulins and autoimmune anti-immunoglobulin antibodies which precipitate in cold serum. They do not occur in normal serum and the globulin is of the IgG, IgA or IgM class. They are found in a variety of chronic infectious diseases such as leprosy and syphilis, in myelomatosis and systemic lupus erythematosus. Their presence should be suspected if an individual suffering from any of these conditions exhibits Raynaud's phenomenon.

4. True

The discovery of antibodies against DNA and nucleoprotein is an important diagnostic feature of systemic lupus erythematosus. In this condition circulating immune complexes may cause glomerulonephritis, arthritis or uveitis whereas in discoid lupus antinuclear antibodies (ANA) are found.

5. False

Circulating immune complexes containing antinuclear antibodies may be found on or eluted from the basement membrane of the renal glomeruli. The resulting damage caused by the complexes finally leads to severe renal insufficiency. In addition to antigen and antibody, deposits of complement components particularly C3 may also occur.

7.8 The germinal centres of lymph nodes:

1. participate in cell-mediated immunity
2. contain macrophages and plasma cells
3. originate in primary follicles
4. enlarge in chronic infectious diseases
5. are absent from the lymph nodes of mice subjected to thymectomy in the neonatal period and in children suffering from the Di George syndrome

1. False

The germinal centres are not concerned with the production of cells concerned with cell-mediated immunity. They are formed in lymph follicles containing B-lymphocytes even in T-lymphocyte depleted animals and they are chiefly concerned with humoral antibody production, developing within the primary nodules of lymphoid tissue in response to an antigenic stimulus.

2. True
In addition to proliferating B-lymphocytes occasional plasma cells of B-lymphocyte origin can be found. In addition macrophages can be seen which contain tingible bodies. These are deeply staining nuclear debris derived from disintegrating cells.

3. True
Primary lymph follicles in the periphery of the lymph nodes are of B-cell origin. These are the site in which the germinal centres form in response to a primary antigenic stimulus. In secondary and subsequent responses germinal centres may form throughout the lymph node.

4. True
In chronic infections lymph node enlargement is common because the nodes respond to a number of antigens. In such an enlarged node a characteristic feature is the number of large germinal centres scattered throughout the lymphoid tissue.

5. False
As germinal centres are of B-lymphocyte origin, their formation is not affected in situations where T-lymphocytes are depleted such as by neonatal thymectomy, or in babies born with Di George syndrome. The Di George syndrome, which is due to failure of development of the third and fourth branchial arches is associated with an absence of the thymus and parathyroid glands.

7.9 Lymphokines, soluble factors released from primed lymphocytes in contact with an antigen are important in:

1. anaphylaxis
2. immune complex disease
3. macrophage activation
4. macrophage migratory inhibition
5. lymphocyte mitogenesis

1. False
This type of reaction is caused by the release of

histamine and other vasoactive substances following a reaction between an antigen and IgE antibody.

2. False
Immune complex diseases are mediated by antigen-antibody complexes causing illnesses such as serum sickness and glomerulonephritis.

3. True
Macrophage activation indicates that these cells have developed an enhanced ability to take part in phagocytosis and eliminate infecting organisms.

4. True
Macrophage migratory inhibition can be demonstrated by packing macrophages and lymphocytes into a capillary tube which is then incubated overnight in a tissue culture medium. In the absence of lymphokines the macrophages migrate from the end of the tube but if lymphokines are present migration is inhibited.

5. True
Lymphocyte mitogenesis indicates that a substance such as a lymphokine causes lymphocyte transformation or mitosis.

7.10 Antibodies may be detected *in vitro* by:

1. precipitation
2. complement fixation
3. lymphokine production
4. lymphocyte transformation test
5. radioimmunoassay

1. True
In many cases, if the concentration of antigen and antibody is high enough, the immune complex will precipitate out of solution, this is the basis of the precipitin test. Precipitation, however, only occurs when the concentration of both antigen and antibody are in 'optimum proportions'. If antigen or antibody is present in excess both remain in solution. Alternatively, if the reagents are placed opposite each other in wells made in an agar plate (Ouchterlony plate) lines of precipitation appear. The basis of immuno-

electrophoresis is also the precipitation of immune complexes in a gel.

2. True

Complement is fixed by immune complexes containing IgM and some subclasses of IgG (IgG1 and IgG3); that fixation of complement has occurred can be detected by adding an indicator system. This may consist of sheep erythrocytes and rabbit (or horse) anti-sheep erythrocyte serum. If lysis of the sheep erythrocytes occurs this indicates that complement is available and has not been fixed by the primary system. Alternatively, if the erythrocytes are not lysed complement has been fixed. This is the basis of several diagnostic tests including the Wassermann reaction for syphilis and the gonococcal complement fixation test for gonorrhoea. Complement fixation tests are also used for the diagnosis of a number of viral infections.

3. False

Lymphokine is produced mainly by T-lymphocytes in cell mediated immune reactions. It is commonly assayed using its migration inhibitory property. In experimental animals peritoneal macrophages and in man buffy coat leucocytes are used for this purpose.

4. False

The lymphocyte transformation test is based on the proliferative response of specifically sensitized T-lymphocytes to an antigen or of T-lymphocytes to mitogens such as phytohaemagglutinin or concanavalin-A. It is, therefore, a test of cell-mediated immunity. The proliferative response is assessed by the incorporation of the radioactive nucleoside ^{3}H-thymidine into the cell DNA.

5. True

IgE antibodies are detected by the radioallergosorbent test (RAST). The antibody is first bound to a solid phase coupled allergen and the bound antibodies are then detected by their ability to bind ^{125}I-labelled immunosorbent-purified antibodies to IgE. Radioimmunoassays are also used to detect antigens such as insulin and haptens such as steroids, thyroid hormones and a number of different drugs.

7.11 Hypogammaglobulinaemia may occur in the following conditions:

1. Prematurity
2. Gluten sensitivity enteropathy
3. Di George syndrome
4. Autoimmune thyroiditis
5. Hodgkin's lymphoma

1. True
Secondary hypogammaglobulinaemia can occur in premature babies. It can be distinguished from hereditary hypogammaglobulinaemia by an estimation of the various gammaglobulin fractions. In premature infants the levels of IgA and IgM are normal whereas in congenital X-linked hypogammaglobulinaemia all five immunoglobulin classes are affected and symptoms begin between 4 and 12 months of life.

2. True
Gluten sensitive enteropathy is associated with secondary hypogammaglobulinaemia. This is believed to be due to the loss of immunoglobin producing cells, i.e. plasma cells, from the disordered gastrointestinal tract.

3. False
The Di George syndrome is not associated with hypogammaglobulinaemia. This condition is due to a defect in the third and fourth branchial arches during embryonic development. It is not, however, genetically controlled. Thymic dysplasia occurs accompanied by an absence of the parathyroid glands. Humoral antibodies are, therefore, normal in concentration but cell-mediated immunity is defective.

4. False
Autoimmune thyroiditis is associated with an increase in the gammaglobulin levels due to the appearance of a variety of antibodies in the circulation. These react against thyroglobulin, the cytoplasmic components of the thyroid and in approximately 6 per cent of patients the gastric parietal cells.

5. True
Secondary hypogammaglobulinaemia occurs in

Hodgkin's disease, lymphosarcoma, chronic lymphatic leukaemia and tumours of the thymus. Low levels of IgG may also be found in multiple myelomatosis because the neoplastic plasma cells are producing abnormal immunoglobulins.

7.12 Active immunity can be produced by an appropriate vaccine to the following diseases:

1. Pneumococcal pneumonia
2. Plague
3. Chicken pox
4. Poliomyelitis
5. Typhoid

1. False
An individual cannot be protected by a vaccine from pneumococcal infections because of the large number of antigenic types within the species.

2. True
If a vaccine is prepared from the prevalent infecting organism a high degree of protection can be achieved. It is, however, of short duration and revaccination is required within a few months.

3. False
Humoral antibodies play little part in virus infections such as chicken pox and mumps. Children suffering from hypogammaglobulinaemia readily recover from such infections even though they rapidly succumb to bacterial infections.

4. True
Live attenuated polio virus which can be administered easily and cheaply by mouth is now the most common method of producing immunity to the polio viruses. In the United Kingdom the trivalent oral vaccine is given at three separate intervals. Between the first and second dose is an interval of 6 to 8 weeks and between the second and third an interval of 4 to 6 months.

5. True
The vaccine most commonly employed consists of a mixture of cultures of *Salmonella typhi* and *Salmonella*

paratyphi A, B and C, killed by heating at about 60°C and preserved in 0.5 per cent phenol.

7.13 The Arthus reaction:

1. is associated with marked emigration of polymorphonuclear leucocytes into the surrounding tissues
2. is not associated with complement activation
3. is a delayed hypersensitivity reaction
4. is associated with vascular damage
5. is produced by endotoxin

1. True
Classically one of the major features of the Arthus reaction is the marked polymorphonuclear infiltrate which occurs at the height of the reaction. Contrast this with the infiltrate of mononuclear cells which accompanies the tuberculin and other forms of delayed hypersensitivity reaction. This polymorphonuclear infiltrate is caused by the local release of C3a and C5a chemotactic factors.

Following the peak of the reaction which occurs after 4 to 8 hours the infiltrate at the site of the reaction becomes progressively more mononuclear.

2. False
The Arthus reaction is due to complement activation which is brought about by the formation of immune complexes from the interaction of antigen with IgG or IgM antibody. Fixation of complement leads to the production of C3a and C5a, otherwise known as anaphylatoxins which bring about the acute inflammatory changes characteristic of this reaction.

3. False
The Arthus reaction is not cell-mediated. It is an immediate hypersensitivity reaction and not due to delayed hypersensitivity. The reaction reaches its maximum intensity between 4 and 8 hours compared to the tuberculin reaction which is maximal between 24 and 48 hours.

4. True
One of the histological features of the Arthus reaction is the damage to the walls of small blood vessels

particularly the venules. This gives rise to the central haemorrhage and necrosis seen in the local reaction.

5. False
Endotoxin activates the alternative pathway of complement, not the classical pathway activated by the immune complexes. The intradermal injection of a sublethal dose of endotoxin produces a non-specific inflammatory reaction with a similar time course to the Arthus reaction. If this is then followed by an intravenous injection some 24 hours later a haemorrhagic reaction develops at the site of the first injection. This is known as the local Schwartzmann reaction.

7.14 Immune complex disease may be associated with:

1. hepatitis B infection
2. skin graft rejection
3. Henoch–Schönlein disease
4. meningococcal infection
5. penicillin therapy

1. True
Hepatitis B is due to a virus. A soluble antigen known as HBsAg (Australia antigen), may be detected in the circulation by precipitation methods in gel or by radioimmunoassay. Polyarteritis nodosa may develop in this type of viral infection when HBsAg, IgM, IgG and C3 is found deposited in vessel walls.

2. False
Immune complexes play no part in skin graft rejection which in man is T-cell mediated. The reaction seen in graft rejection is similar to the tuberculin reaction.

3. True
Acute haemorrhagic glomerulonephritis of immune complex origin may occur in children. It is chiefly associated with streptococcal infection although the high titres of anti-streptolysin O found in rheumatic fever are not found. Acute cutaneous vasculitis leading to a purpuric rash, together with haemorrhage

and serosanguineous effusion into the gut may also occur.

4. True
Meningococcal infection may be associated with certain stigmata of immune complex disease, such as cutaneous vasculitis, arthritis, and episcleritis. Immunoglobulin and complement have been detected in the walls of the cutaneous vessels and the synovium.

5. True
Penicillin therapy is frequently associated with evidence of both anaphylactic and immune complex sensitivity. The development of a papular or morbilliform rash, arthritis and transient proteinuria are evidence supporting the presence of immune complex disease.

7.15 The third component of complement is:

1. a factor in phagocytosis
2. an anaphylatoxin
3. chemotactic
4. migration inhibition factor
5. an interferon

1. True
The so-called non-specific opsonin is mainly C3 produced by C3 convertase. Activation of C3 may occur as the result of immune complexes via the classical pathway, or by endotoxin and related polysaccharides through the alternative pathway. Complement is important in the opsonisation of bacteria and other foreign matter through the heat-labile C3b product which coating the micro-organisms and other antigenic particles facilitates their phagocytosis.

2. True
An anaphylatoxin is a substance produced during the fixation of complement which causes the release of histamine from tissue mast cells. Anaphylatoxin activity is present in C3a and C5a fractions of complement. An assay of anaphylatoxin activity can be made by observing the contraction of plain muscle in a Schultz–Dale bath. Anaphylatoxin release is be-

lieved to be the cause of the local oedema in the Arthus reaction.

3. True
C3a and C5a are chemotactic to polymorphonuclear leucocytes. This explains the intense polymorphonuclear infiltration which occurs in the Arthus reaction or following the intradermal injection of endotoxin.

4. False
Migration inhibitory factor (MIF) is a lymphokine released by the activation of T-lymphocytes by an antigen or mitogen. The target cell is usually a macrophage. However, this factor can also be assayed on human buffy coat leucocytes.

5. False
Interferon is an antiviral agent released by a wide range of cells including lymphocytes. It is non-specifically produced following stimulation of tissue cells by a wide range of viruses, or from lymphocytes by the action of mitogens or antigens if the lymphocytes have been specifically sensitised. It has been classified as a lymphokine but it is not related to classical lymphokines such as MIF, mitogenic factor or lymphotoxin.

7.16 Anaphylaxis:

1. develops 24 hours after the initial stimulus
2. causes an urticarial eruption
3. is produced by IgA antibody
4. causes eosinophilia
5. causes degranulation of basophils and mast cells

1. False
Anaphylaxis is mediated by an antigen interacting with IgE on the surface of the mast cells. This causes a very rapid degranulation of such cells which is accompanied by a massive local and systemic release of vasoactive amines including histamine. A reaction either local or general can, therefore, frequently be seen within 5 minutes.

2. True
The local release of histamine from the mast cells causes capillary dilatation, an increase in their permeability and contraction of smooth muscle. This

increase in capillary permeability in the skin is the cause of the urticarial rash.

3. False
Anaphylaxis is caused by sensitisation of the mast cells by IgE which, when exposed again to the appropriate antigen, become degranulated. IgA is the antibody type produced by the mucus surfaces of the gut, respiratory tract and urinary tract. It is mainly antimicrobial and protective.

4. True
The eosinophil chemotactic factor of anaphylaxis (ECF-A) is released following interaction between antigen and specific IgE antibody. It should also be noted that the formation of IgE is particularly stimulated in parasitic infections causing the eosinophilia so characteristically seen in nematode worm infestations.

5. True
Degranulation of basophils and mast cells follows the interaction between an antigen and IgE. These granules contain heparin and it is this which stains metachromatically with toluidine blue. The histamine which these cells contain is formed from histidine by the enzyme histidine decarboxylase but in addition to histamine, 5-hydroxytryptamine (serotonin), the slow reacting substance of anaphylaxis (SRS-A) and basophil kallikrein may be released. The latter cleaves the plasma euglobulin kininogen to kinins. The release of these pharmacologically active agents causes local phenomena to develop. These include conjunctivitis, rhinorrhoea, laryngeal oedema, asthma, angioneurotic oedema and urticaria. The systemic effects of such agents include the dilatation of the mesenteric vessels, hypotension, tachycardia and finally shock.

7.17 Complement activation takes place:

1. in the presence of endotoxin
2. as part of the tuberculin reaction
3. by more than one pathway
4. in anaphylaxis
5. by antigen IgA interaction

1. True
Endotoxins, certain bacterial and other polysaccharides activate complement by their interaction with an initiating factor (IF). Complement activation then takes place via the alternative pathway which bypasses C1, C4 and C2. This pathway involves properdin which is a non-immunoglobulin gammaglobulin and factor B, otherwise known as C3 proactivator. Properdin itself is considered to act as a stabiliser of the C3b–Factor B complex.

2. False
The tuberculin reaction does not involve the complement system. It is a delayed hypersensitivity reaction in which the pharmacological mediators are lymphokines.

3. True
There are at least three pathways to C3.
  (a) Classical conversion—immune complexes via C1, C4 and C2
  (b) The alternative pathway—endotoxin and polysaccharides via Factor B and properdin
  (c) Plasminogen pathway via the Hageman factor

4. False
Anaphylaxis does not involve the complement cascade but is mediated by the interaction of IgE with the mast cells which then release vasoactive amines including histamine. This mechanism must not be confused with the action of anaphylatoxin which is the result of C3 activation and the production of C3a and C5a. Anaphylatoxin when injected into animals produces an anaphylactic reaction with the release of histamine but without the intervention of IgE.

5. False
Although aggregated IgA can activate the alternative pathway under rare experimental conditions, it is considered that antigen IgA interaction does not normally work through the classical complement cascade.

7.18 The production of antibody is essential to host resistance in the following infection:

1. Leprosy
2. Pneumococcal pneumonia

3. Vaccinia
4. Tetanus
5. Malaria

1. False
Host resistance to infection with the *Mycobacterium leprae* is cell-mediated. Patients suffering from the tuberculoid form of the disease have positive lepromin tests and *in vitro* evidence of strong cell-mediated immunity. Contrast this with lepromatous leprosy in which patients are unable to eliminate the *M. leprae* which are found in huge numbers in the macrophages. These latter patients have high levels of anti-mycobacterial antibody, negative lepromin tests and negative *in vitro* tests of cell-mediated immunity. Lepromatous leprosy can, therefore, be considered to be due to a specific failure of cell-mediated immunity which results in a patient being unable to eliminate the organism.

2. True
Prior to the introduction of sulphonamides and antibiotics serotherapy was effectively used in the treatment of pneumococcal infections.

3. False
Children suffering from T-cell deficiency, the Di George syndrome, develop a disseminated vaccinial infection when they are vaccinated. Children with a pure B-cell deficiency which is associated with a total inability to produce immunoglobin can, in contrast, be vaccinated without harmful effects.

4. True
Tetanus antitoxin is used in the treatment of tetanus although if it is prepared in species other than man it may give rise to severe and fatal anaphylaxis. The best means of avoiding the complications associated with infection by *Cl. tetani* is prophylactic immunisation with tetanus toxoid, which results in a high level of circulating antibody.

5. True
There is no evidence that host resistance to the plasmodia is cell-mediated. Hyperimmune globulin has been shown effective in this infection although there is no effective vaccine capable of increasing the resistance of man to infection with these protozoa.

7.19 Serum sickness

1. can be caused by an injection of diphtheria anti-toxin
2. is caused by the injection of tetanus toxoid
3. is caused by the injection of penicillin
4. may be immune complex mediated
5. may be anaphylactic

1. True
Serum sickness may develop in individuals passively immunised with diphtheria antitoxin prepared in the horse. If the individual has not been previously sensitised by administration of the heterologous serum an acute generalised reaction occurs within 7 to 10 days of the injection. If previously sensitised the reaction occurs much sooner.

2. False
Tetanus toxoid is used for the active immunisation of individuals in order to protect them against infections with *Clostridium tetani*. It is a formolised preparation of tetanus toxin which although immunogenic is not allergenic. It does not give rise to IgE anaphylactic antibodies or induce immune complex disease.

3. True
Allergic reactions to penicillin are relatively common, the hypersensitivity being directed towards the penicilloyl (degradation) residue. Such reactions may give rise to a chronic syndrome taking the form of a cutaneous eruption, arthritis or proteinuria.

4. True
Immune complex disease is the cause of chronic serum sickness. It may cause glomerulonephritis, arthritis, uveitis and cutaneous vasculitis due to the deposition of immune complexes (IgG or IgM), and complement on, for example, the glomerular basement membrane or synovial surfaces.

5. True
Acute serum sickness, due to IgE antibody reacting with antigen on the mast cell surface, may give rise to anaphylactic shock, angioneurotic oedema, laryngeal oedema or acute bronchospasm.

165

7.20 Anaphylactic reactions commonly follow the administration of the following drugs:

1. Penicillin
2. Azathioprine
3. Procaine
4. Alpha methyl-dopa
5. Hydralazine

1. True
Penicillin is an important cause of anaphylactic reactions. The penicilloyl degradation product acts as an hapten binding onto body protein, inducing the formation of IgE antibodies.

2. False
Azathioprine is an immunosuppressive drug used in renal transplantation and for the treatment of some immune complex diseases such as systemic lupus erythematosus. It is an analogue of guanine and acts as a false base when incorporated into DNA.

3. True
Procaine can act as a hapten binding to protein to become antigenic.

4. False
One toxic side effect of α-methyldopa is the production of a Coombs positive haemolytic anaemia. The antigen to which the antibodies are directed has rhesus specificity and there is no immune response to the drug as such.

5. False
Hydralazine is one cause of drug induced systemic lupus erythematosus. The antibody induced is an antinuclear factor, and the resulting disease is due to immune complexes.

7.21 An autoimmune haemolytic anaemia:

1. does not occur in systemic lupus erythematosus
2. does not show rhesus specificity
3. may be associated with mycoplasma infection
4. may be caused by drug therapy
5. is not associated with leucopenia

1. False
Autoantibodies to erythrocytes, leucocytes and platelets commonly occur in systemic lupus erythematosus. In addition a number of other immunological abnormalities can be found. They include antinuclear factors, high immunoglobulin levels and antigen-antibody complexes.

2. False
In 30 per cent of patients suffering from a haemolytic anaemia due to 'warm autoantibodies', the specificity of some of these is directed to one or more of the rhesus antibodies, commonly anti-c or anti-e.

3. True
Haemolytic anaemia associated with 'cold autoantibodies' showing specificity for the I antigen, can occur in infections due to *Mycoplasma pulmonis*.

4. True
Drugs which may be associated with an autoimmune haemolytic anaemia include p-amino salicylic acid, phenacetin, quinidine, quinine, chlorpromazine and penicillin, as well as α-methyldopa.

5. False
Haemolytic anaemia is commonly associated with both a leucopenia and thrombocytopenia. Autoimmune pancytopenia may result from drug therapy as well as occurring in systemic lupus erythematosus.

7.22 The following are, or contain, autoantibodies:

1. Cryoglobulins
2. Rheumatoid factor
3. Migration inhibitory factor
4. Antinuclear factor
5. Transfer factor

1. True
Cryoglobulins are immune complexes formed by the reaction between immunoglobulins and anti-immunoglobulin antibodies. Characteristically they precipitate after overnight storage in the refrigerator or when serum is cooled below 37°C. Cryoglobulins are present in the plasma in a wide range of chronic infections and autoimmune diseases, including systemic lupus erythematosus.

2. True

Rheumatoid factor is an IgM anti-immunoglobulin antibody with specificity directed against the Gm groups on the Fc portion of immunoglobulin molecules. It can be detected by the agglutination of latex particles coated with immunoglobulin or by the agglutination of sheep erythrocytes that have reacted with specific rabbit immunoglobulin (Rose Waaler test). This factor is found in the sera of patients with rheumatoid arthritis and is valuable in distinguishing this disease from the polyarthritis associated with psoriasis. It may also occur, however, in the sera of patients suffering from chronic infections or chronic autoimmune disease.

3. False

The migration inhibitory factor is a lymphokine produced by the action of an antigen or mitogen on T-lymphocytes. It inhibits the migration from capillary tubes, *in vitro*, of macrophages obtained from a peritoneal exudate or leucocytes from the human buffy coat from capillary tubes *in vitro*.

4. True

The antinuclear factor is an autoantibody directed against DNA and nucleoproteins. It is present in the sera of patients suffering from systemic lupus erythematosus. It may also occur in the sera of patients suffering from chronic infectious diseases such as leprosy and in connective tissue diseases such as Sjögren's syndrome.

5. False

Transfer factor is an extract of human buffy coat leucocytes that can transfer tuberculin sensitivity and other delayed hypersensitivity reactions.

7.23 Antiglobulins may be involved in the:

1. Wassermann reaction
2. Coombs test
3. fluorescent antibody test
4. rheumatoid factor test
5. Casoni test

1. False

The Wassermann reaction is a complement fixation

test in which the antigen is cardiolipin derived from ox heart with which the antibody, probably an autoantibody developing in syphilis, reacts. The indicator system used consists of sheep erythrocytes and rabbit (or horse) anti-sheep erythrocyte antibody.

2. True
The direct Coombs test is an agglutination reaction in which erythrocytes coated with antibody are agglutinated by an antiglobulin reagent. The direct Coombs test indicates that sensitised erythrocytes are already present in the circulation as occurs in some haemolytic anaemias. In the indirect test the red cells are sensitised in the laboratory by antibody before exposure to the antiglobulin reagent. This is a very sensitive test for non-agglutinating rhesus antibodies in a patient's serum.

3. True
In the direct fluorescent antibody test fluoroscein may be linked to an antiglobulin through an isothiocyanate linkage. This is then used to detect the presence of bound immunoglobulin fixed in the tissue. Antinuclear factor and other autoantibodies, such as antimitochondrial or antimicrosomal antibodies can be detected by this means.

4. True
Rheumatoid factor is an IgM anti-immunoglobulin molecule that binds to the Gm groups on the Fc portion of the immunoglobulin molecules. It may be detected by the latex agglutination test or Rose Waaler test (see 9.11). The highest concentrations are found in rheumatoid arthritis.

5. False
The Casoni test is used for the diagnosis of hydatid disease, the causal agent of which is the *Echinococcus granulosus*. In a patient suffering from hydatid disease a local anaphylactic reaction occurs within 15 minutes of the injection of hydatid antigen into the skin with the development of a flare followed by a weal.

7.24 Cell mediated immunity involves the following mechanisms:

1. IgG

2. T-lymphocytes
3. Eosinophil leucocytes
4. Complement
5. Macrophages

1. False
IgG is an immunoglobulin which is involved only in humoral immunity.

2. True
T-lymphocytes, lymphocytes derived from the thymus, play a major role in cell mediated immunity. In addition they are also concerned in the production of humoral immunity because they release factors which augment the action of the B-lymphocytes.

3. False
Eosinophils play no part in cell mediated immunity. They are concerned in immediate hypersensitivity reactions. They are also found in greater than normal numbers in the circulation of patients infested with nematodes (worms).

4. False
Complement is an enzymatic system of serum proteins activated by many antigen-antibody reactions.

5. True
Macrophages act as carriers of antigen to the lymphoid tissue. They are also the most important non-specific effector cells in cell-mediated immune reactions.

7.25 The following tests are based upon the delayed hypersensitivity reaction:

1. Schick test
2. Pseudo-Schick test
3. Frei test
4. Leishmanin test
5. Prausnitz–Kustner reaction

1. False
The Schick test is used to determine an individual's susceptibility to infection with *Corynebacterium diphtheriae*, the causative organism of diphtheria. The test consists of the intradermal injection of a small

dose of diphtheria exotoxin. If an inflammatory reaction develops at the site of the injection reaching its maximum intensity within 4 to 7 days the individual is susceptible to the toxin and hence vulnerable to the disease. A negative test indicates the presence of antitoxin in the circulation. As a control a similar quantity of purified toxoid should be inoculated into the other forearm.

2. True
The Pseudo-Schick test is a delayed hypersensitivity reaction which occurs in response to the intradermal injection of both diphtheria toxoid or toxin. The maximum intensity of this reaction is generally reached before 48 hours. This reaction leads to difficulties in the interpretation of the Schick test.

3. True
The Frei test is a delayed hypersensitivity reaction which is used for the diagnosis of lymphogranuloma venereum. This disease is caused by an organism of the chlamydia group which is 250 to 300 nm in diameter. They are, therefore, larger than virus particles but smaller than bacteria. A suspension of the organisms intradermally injected in a patient suffering from the disease gives rise to an indurated erythematous papule 4 days later. Chlamydia are also responsible for psittacosis and trachoma.

4. True
The Leishmanin test is a delayed hypersensitivity reaction which is used for the diagnosis of cutaneous leishmaniasis, oriental sore. This condition is caused by *Leishmania tropica*. This test is negative in the more generalised form of leishmaniasis caused by *L. donovani*, known as kala-azar, although both the parasites are morphologically identical. The vector in both diseases is the sandfly, genus *Phlebotomus*.

5. False
The Prausnitz–Kustner reaction is not a delayed hypersensitivity reaction. It takes its name from the two investigators who first demonstrated the presence of an antibody-like factor termed reagin in the serum of atopic individuals, i.e. individuals who have a constitutional or hereditary tendency to develop immediate hypersensitivity states such as asthma or hay fever to allergens which would pro-

voke no reaction in normal subjects. The reaction is provoked by intradermally injecting the serum of a patient with IgE antibody then making a prick test with an allergen at the same site 24 hours later. The reaction is a weal and flare within 15 minutes. This test should not be used because of the risk of transmitting hepatitis B virus.

7.26 The following are the chief characteristics of delayed hypersensitivity reactions:

1. The development of a polymorphonuclear leucocyte infiltrate
2. The reaction has reached its maximum intensity at 4 hours
3. An individual can be passively sensitised with serum
4. It is associated with increased T-lymphocyte function
5. Complement activation is an essential feature

1. False
Delayed hypersensitivity reactions in man are associated with infiltrates of mononuclear cells, chiefly lymphocytes and macrophages.

2. False
Delayed hypersensitivity reactions are maximal in primed subjects 24 to 48 hours after challenge. This compares with Arthus reactions which develop as a result of the union of antigen and free antibody with the subsequent activation (fixation) of complement. Such a reaction is maximal at 4 hours.

3. False
Delayed hypersensitivity reactions are not antibody mediated and, therefore, passive sensitisation with serum is impossible. In experimental systems delayed hypersensitivity can be transferred by the use of lymphocyte suspensions obtained from the peripheral blood, lymph nodes or spleen.

4. True
Delayed hypersensitivity follows interaction between specifically sensitised T-lymphocytes and antigen, the result of which is the release of lymphokine which then acts mainly on macrophages.

172

Delayed hypersensitivity is associated with T-lymphocyte proliferation in the paracortical or thymus dependent areas of lymph nodes and spleen.

5. False

Complement is not involved in the mechanisms of delayed hypersensitivity. The equivalent non-specific mediator is lymphokine which is the generic name given to a number of soluble factors, mainly glycoproteins with a molecular weight of 40 000 which are released from the activated T-lymphocytes and whose chief target cell is the macrophage.

7.27 Maximum changes occur in the following skin reactions within 24 to 48 hours:

1. Schwartzmann reaction
2. Arthus reaction
3. Tuberculin reaction
4. Contact patch test
5. Skin allograft rejection

1. False

The Schwartzmann reaction is a haemorrhagic reaction in the skin or tissues which reaches its maximum within 4 hours. The local Schwartzmann reaction is elicited in the following manner: an intradermal injection of endotoxin or related polysaccharide is administered followed 24 hours later by an intravenous injection. A generalised reaction involving particularly the lungs and kidneys can be produced if both doses of endotoxin are administered intravenously. It is considered by many investigators that this haemorrhagic reaction underlies similar phenomena observed in bacterial infections such as meningococcal infections in which haemorrhagic destruction of the adrenal glands results in the development of the Waterhouse–Friedrichsen syndrome.

2. False

The Arthus reaction which is the result of union between antigen and free antibody with the subsequent activation of complement reaches a maximum between 4 and 8 hours. The reaction is chiefly associated with accumulation of polymorphonuclear leucocytes and the aggregation of platelets. Macroscopically the reaction is oedematous and haemor-rhagic due to local vasculitis.

3. True
The tuberculin reaction is the prototype of all delayed hypersensitivity reactions. This reaction reaches a maximum in 48 hours in man, but may reach its peak earlier in experimental animals. It is delayed in time because it is a T-cell mediated reaction and this period is required for the macro-phages to accumulate at the site of antigen deposi-tion.

4. True
Contact sensitivity reactions—patch tests used in dermatological practice—are also delayed hypersen-sitivity reactions to antigens fixed in the periphery. The small molecular weight chemical sensitiser binds to epidermal proteins by covalent linkages and thus acts as a hapten.

5. False
Although the rejection of a skin graft is also a T-cell mediated immune phenomenon, approximately 10 days are required for rejection. This is because on primary graft application, it is necessary for the graft to heal and establish a blood supply from the host after which the primary immune response develops. This has a latent period of at least 5 days.

7.28 Cell-mediated immune processes are of great importance in the control of the following infec-tions:

1. Pneumococcal pneumonia
2. Diphtheria
3. Tuberculosis
4. Candidiasis
5. Mumps

1. False
Cell-mediated immunity plays no part in the host's defences against pneumococcal infections. These organisms are opsonised and killed by humoral antibody and complement. The specificity of the antibody is directed against the 'specific soluble substance', the pneumococcal polysaccharide. Anti-

bodies against these soluble antigens were used prior to the introduction of antibiotics for immunotherapeutic purposes with some success.

2. False

Cell mediated immunity is not involved in diphtheritic infections. *Corynebacterium diptheriae* is harmful because it produces an exotoxin which particularly damages the myocardium and peripheral nerves. This toxin may be inactivated before it is fixed in the tissues by an antitoxin which can be prepared in the horse. The use of this antitoxin carries the risk of anaphylaxis or serum sickness and, therefore, active immunisation with toxoid is preferable.

3. True

Host resistance to mycobacteria is dependent on cell-mediated immune processes. The mycobacteria are facultative intracellular parasites and are found mainly within macrophages. If cell-mediated immunity fails dissemination of the disease occurs and frequently a negative delayed hypersensitivity test is found as in miliary tuberculosis.

4. True

A failure of cell-mediated immunity is frequently associated with mucocutaneous or diffuse candidiasis. Thus diffuse candidiasis may occur in Hodgkin's disease and non-Hodgkin's lymphomas and in the primary T-cell deficiencies of childhood associated with a specific failure of T-cell response to candida antigens. Transfer factor has been successfully used to treat muco-cutaneous candidiasis by specifically increasing the T-cell response to *Candida albicans*.

5. True

Mumps is caused by a paramyxovirus. Previous infection with mumps virus is associated with a positive delayed hypersensitivity skin reaction. Mumps antigen is one of the standard skin test reagents used to diagnose a general non-specific loss of cell-mediated immunity in adults with conditions such as non-Hodgkin's lymphomas, Hodgkin's disease and sarcoidosis.

7.29 The following micro-organisms are obligate or falcultative intracellular parasites:

1. *Mycobacterium tuberculosis*

2. *Clostridium welchii*
3. *Corynebacterium diphtheriae*
4. *Leishmania tropica*
5. Herpes simplex

1. True
M. tuberculosis may be found within macrophages or other cells of the mononuclear phagocyte series in the centre of a typical epithelioid cell granuloma. *Myco. tuberculosis* requires active cell-mediated immune processes for its elimination.

2. False
Cl. welchii, one of the organisms involved in gas gangrene, is protected from the body's defence mechanisms because it is an anaerobic spore bearing organism. The clostridia produce tissue damage by means of exotoxins which are proteolytic and saccharolytic enzymes. In addition the organism produces hyaluronidase which breaks down tissue barriers, thus enabling the organisms to spread through the connective tissue planes. Protection from the clostridial group of organisms may be obtained by the use of an anti gas gangrene serum.

3. False
C. diphtheriae is an aerobic bacillus usually found extracellularly. Its effects are produced by an exotoxin affecting the myocardium and peripheral nerves which can be neutralised by a specific antitoxin.

4. True
The amastigote form of *L. tropica*, the causative organism of oriental sore, is generally found within macrophages in a granuloma lying within the dermis. In this form the organisms are referred to as 'Leishman-donovan' bodies.

5. True
Herpes simplex is caused by a virus of the herpes virus group. This group also includes varicella/zoster, the Epstein–Barr virus and cytomegalovirus. Herpes infections are recurrent with long latent periods. Prior to the eruption the virus remains latent in the cells of the posterior root ganglia.

7.30 The following tests may be used to assess host resistance in mycobacterial infections:

1. Skin tests
2. Complement fixation
3. Lymphocyte transformation test
4. Radioimmunoassay
5. Leucocyte migration inhibition test

1. True
The classical way of assessing whether a patient has had previous contact with the *Mycobacterium tuberculosis* and hence has developed some resistance by means of cell-mediated immunity to the disease is by the tuberculin test. A positive test is indicated by the development over 18 to 48 hours of an inflammatory indurated response in the skin into which tuberculin has been injected. This test is negative during the early stages of infection and in rapidly progressive forms of the disease, e.g. miliary tuberculosis. Similarly the lepromin test conducted with a suspension of *Mycobacterium leprae* is positive in tuberculoid leprosy and in normal adults but is negative in lepromatous leprosy in which the tissues team with organisms.

2. False
Complement fixation tests are basically used to assess antibody production and since host resistance to mycobacterial infections is cell-mediated these tests play no part in estimating such resistance. Complement fixation tests are used in the diagnosis of viral infections and some bacterial infections such as gonorrhoea and syphilis.

3. True
In this test the patient's lymphocytes are incubated with a mitogen such as phytohaemagglutinin or an antigen to which they have been primed for some 3 to 5 days. If positive the cells become transformed into large blast cells which readily incorporate ^{3}H-thymidine. This test is used as an *in vitro* correlate of delayed hypersensitivity and as such frequently correlates well with resistance to infection in conditions in which T-cells are important in host protection.

4. False
Radioimmunoassay is used to measure specific IgE

antibodies to allergens such as pollens in the RAST (radioallergosorbent test). It can also be used to measure the concentration of hormones such as insulin in the blood if a specific antiserum is available.

5. True
Buffy coat leucocytes can, under normal circumstances, if cultured overnight, be induced to grow out of the ends of capillary tubes in a fan-like manner. In the presence of antigen and specifically sensitised T-lymphocytes, however, migration is inhibited by lymphokine. Such migration inhibition correlates with delayed hypersensitivity and host resistance in mycobacterial infections.

7.31 The following cells play an important role in skin allograft rejection:

1. Polymorphonuclear leucocytes
2. Macrophages
3. Mast cells
4. B-lymphocytes
5. T-lymphocytes

1. False
Polymorphonuclear leucocytes play no part in skin allograft rejection. These cells play their major role in acute inflammatory reactions and immunological reactions mediated by immune complex deposition, such as the Arthus reaction.

2. True
Skin allograft rejection is a T-cell mediated event in which lymphokine is released. The latter is the generic name given to soluble factors released by primed lymphocytes after contact with a specific antigen. These substances are chemotactic for macrophages and cause the activation of macrophage enzymes. Macrophages form the major cellular component of the mononuclear infiltrate which develops around a skin allograft prior to rejection.

3. False
These cells play no part in skin allograft rejection. They are of particular importance, however, in anaphylactic reactions when degranulation results in

the liberation of vasoactive amines, histamine, serotonin, SRS-A and kallikrein. Degranulation is initiated by the interaction between antigen and IgE antibody on the cell membrane.

4. False
The B-lymphocytes are the precursors of plasma cells which produce immunoglobulins. The latter are not considered to play a major role in skin graft rejection. B-lymphocytes, which are not so mobile as T-lymphocytes, are found chiefly in collections in central lymphoid tissues, i.e. the spleen and lymph nodes, particularly in the lymph follicles, germinal centres and at the cortico-medullary junction.

5. True
Skin allograft rejection is a cell-mediated event caused by the reaction of specifically sensitised T-lymphocytes with antigen. The T-lymphocytes are part of the mobile pool of long-lived lymphocytes which may be found circulating through the tissues and in the lymph. They migrate into the tissues particularly through post-capillary venules. The production of lymphokine by reaction with antigen brings the next most important cell, the macrophage, into the area of activity.

7.32 The following substances are lymphokines:

1. Properdin
2. Migration inhibitory factor
3. Macrophage chemotactic factor
4. Factor B
5. Interferon

1. False
Properdin is a β globulin found in normal serum. It is part of the complement alternative pathway to C3 conversion by-passing C1, C4 and C2. It is activated by bacterial endotoxins and polysaccharides such as zymosan which is obtained from yeast and insulin. Mg^{++} but not Ca^{++} ions are necessary for the activation of the alternative pathway.

2. True
The migration inhibitory factor (MIF), a glycoprotein with a molecular weight of approximately 40 000,

179

was the first of the various substances now known under the generic title of lymphokines to be discovered. It is assayed by its ability to inhibit the migration of macrophages obtained from the peritoneal exudate of the guinea-pig from capillary tubes *in vitro*. MIF production is used as a standard *in vitro* correlate of delayed hypersensitivity.

3. True
Macrophage chemotactic factor is another lymphokine. It is distinguished from the polymorph chemotactic factor by its molecular weight. It is assayed by its ability to attract macrophages onto a millipore membrane in a closed Boyden chamber.

4. False
Factor B is an important component in the alternative pathway of complement activation. It is also referred to as C3 proactivator.

5. True
Interferons are a family of substances, molecular weight approximately 30 000, produced by cells infected with a virus or by synthetic inducers such as polyinosinic and polycytidylic acid (poly I:C). They can also be produced by T-lymphocytes activated by antigen or mitogen and as such are included in lists of lymphokines. When taken up by other cells interferon inhibits the replication of virus within them.

7.33 Graft versus host disease:
1. may follow bone marrow transplants
2. may follow blood transfusion
3. occurs in Hodgkin's disease
4. can be suppressed by tetracyclines
5. can be suppressed by cyclophosphamide

1. True
Bone marrow transplants are used as a therapeutic measure in patients suffering from the combined immunodeficiency syndrome or whose immune response has been destroyed by irradiation or cytotoxic drugs. If the marrow transplant is not HLA matched the donor T-lymphocytes will react against host tissues. Signs that this is occurring include the development of erythroderma, exfoliative dermati-

tis, splenomegaly and wasting. Death ultimately occurs if the reaction cannot be controlled by immunosuppressive agents such as cyclosporin A.

2. True
In patients suffering from a severe depression of their immunological systems a blood transfusion may provoke a graft versus host reaction due to the T-cells which are contained in the donor blood. This can be avoided by irradiating the blood prior to transfusion in order to destroy T-cell function.

3. False
Graft versus host disease could only occur in a patient with Hodgkin's disease if that patient was rendered completely immunodeficient by irradiation or cytotoxic therapy and then received a transfusion of unirradiated blood.

4. False
Tetracyclines will only suppress the intercurrent infection that occurs as the graft versus host reaction becomes severe and then only if the bacteria causing the infection are sensitive to this antibiotic. This is not usually the case since the common agents of infection in this disease are fungi and viruses, all of which are insensitive to the tetracyclines.

5. True
Temporary suppression of the graft versus host reaction can be achieved by the use of cyclophosphamide because this drug is a nitrogen mustard derivative cytotoxic to dividing lymphocytes. It is, however, an extremely toxic compound which may cause hair loss resulting in alopecia, destruction of the bladder mucosa causing haematuria and increasing susceptibility to fungal infection.

7.34 The following can cause immunological unresponsiveness:

1. Immunological tolerance
2. Immunological enhancement
3. Freund's adjuvant
4. T-lymphocytes
5. Antigen-antibody complexes

1. True
Immunological tolerance is the term given to the

specific immunological unresponsiveness caused by the elimination or depletion of a specific clone of immunologically competent cells. This may be the result of exposure to high concentrations of antigen, particularly in late fetal or early neonatal life which is the period of immunological immaturity. This phenomenon is mainly applicable to allograft rejection.

2. True
Immunological enhancement paradoxically does not refer to the enhancement of the immune response but to enhancement of tumour growth. This is caused by the stimulation by the tumour of a blocking antibody which combines with the antigenic sites on the surface of the tumour cells. This results in a markedly decreased stimulation of cell mediated immunity against the tumour and also prevents the sensitised T-cells reacting with tumour antigens to kill the tumour cells.

3. False
Freund's adjuvant is a water in oil emulsion with or without added mycobacteria. The addition of antigen to this mixture promotes both increased antibody formation and delayed hypersensitivity.

4. True
A special subpopulation of T-lymphocytes may act as suppressor cells diminishing the immune response. In mice these cells can be distinguished by the presence of surface antigens (Ly antigens) from the effector cells of delayed hypersensitivity and helper cells required both *in vitro* and *in vivo* for antibody formation.

5. True
The presence of soluble antigen-antibody complexes formed between soluble tumour antigens and antibody in the circulation can suppress the cell mediated immune response against tumours and lead to enhanced tumour growth.

7.35 The following infections are common in immunodeficient patients:

1. *Pneumocystis carinii*
2. Diphtheria

3. Poliomyelitis
4. Cytomegalovirus
5. *Candida albicans*

1. True
Pneumocystis carinii is a protozoon related to the plasmodia and toxoplasma. It is ubiquitous in the upper respiratory tract but causes chronic pneumonia in patients who have become immunodeficient whether due to malnutrition, the administration of cytotoxic drugs in the treatment of Hodgkin's disease or primary T-lymphocyte deficiency.

2. False
There is no evidence that an increase in infection by *Corynebacterium diphtheriae* occurs in immunodeficient subjects.

3. False
There is no evidence of an increase in infection with poliovirus occurring in immunodeficient subjects.

4. True
Cytomegalovirus is a herpes virus causing cytomegalic inclusion disease. Although infection with this virus is commonly associated with the newborn it is also an important opportunistic infection occurring in immunodeficient patients. The virus affects many tissues and intracellular inclusion bodies are found particularly in the bronchial epithelium.

5. True
Mucocutaneous candidiasis is a particular complication of immunodeficiency regardless of the cause. It is generally associated with other evidence of depressed T-lymphocyte function, negative candidin skin test, depressed lymphocyte transformation test and absent leucocyte migration inhibition test with candida antigens. Other non-specific tests of T-lymphocyte function may also be depressed.

7.36 The following conditions are associated with T-cell immunodeficiency:

1. Hodgkin's disease
2. Tay–Sachs disease
3. Wiskott Aldrich syndrome
4. Down's syndrome
5. Di George syndrome

1. True
The pathological tissue in Hodgkin's disease permeates the T-lymphocyte areas of lymphoid tissue, the B-lymphocytes and plasma cells remaining unaffected. Many of the tests of T-lymphocyte function (skin tests, mitogen induced lymphocyte transformation) become depressed as the disease progresses. Patients become susceptible to opportunistic infections with organisms normally controlled by T-lymphocyte function, including *Pneumocystis carinii*, cytomegalovirus, *Candida albicans* and other fungal agents.

2. False
Tay–Sachs disease is a lipid storage disease affecting the nervous system only. The ganglion cells are ballooned with ganglioside giving rise to Amaurotic Familial Idiocy. These children typically have a cherry red spot in the macula.

3. True
This is a sex linked recessive disease of childhood characterised by atopic eczema and thrombocytopenia. Failure of T-lymphocyte function occurs as the disease progresses and the children become susceptible to viral, fungal and bacterial infections.

4. False
Down's syndrome, once known as mongolism, is associated with trisomy of chromosome 21. This chromosomal abnormality gives rise to mental retardation as well as the characteristic physical features. Although there may be an increased incidence of leukaemias it is not associated with immunodeficiency.

5. True
The Di George syndrome is due to a defect in development of the third and fourth branchial arches resulting in thymic aplasia and T-cell immunodeficiency, together with an absence of the parathyroid glands which causes hypocalcaemic tetany.

7.37 A non-specific depression of the tuberculin reaction occurs in:

1. influenza
2. measles

3. sarcoidosis
4. leprosy
5. ulcerative colitis

1. False
Infection with the influenza virus does not lead to non-specific depression of cell-mediated immunity.

2. True
The depression of tuberculin reactivity in measles was first described by Von Pirquet in 1908 and it was eventually established that this was the result of infection of the T-lymphocytes with the virus. The disease is frequently accompanied by a lymphopenia. The lymphocyte transformation and leucocyte migration inhibition responses to tuberculin and candida antigens are lost.

3. True
Certain parameters of T-lymphocyte function are depressed in sarcoidosis including the tuberculin reaction and ability to cause sensitisation with 2.4 dinitrochlorobenzene (DNCB). In addition, the lymphocyte transformation response in the presence of phytohaemagglutinin (PHA) may be depressed.

4. True
A non-specific depression of tuberculin reactivity and the ability to be sensitised with DNCB occurs in over 50 per cent of patients with lepromatous leprosy but only occasionally in tuberculoid leprosy. However, there is no generalised decline in T-lymphocyte function which apart from the specific loss of cell-mediated immunity against *Mycobacterium leprae* is otherwise normal.

5. False
There is no evidence of even a partial loss of T-lymphocyte function in ulcerative colitis and tuberculin reactivity remains therefore within normal limits.

7.38 Haptoglobins

1. bind to the body's own proteins to make them immunogenic
2. are immunoglobulins
3. bind to free haemoglobin

4. are controlled by genetic factors
5. can bind rheumatoid factor

1. False
Haptens are simple chemical groupings that are too small to be immunogenic, but can interact with antibody. They can bind to proteins generally by covalent linkages to become immunogenic.

2. False
Haptoglobins are α_2 globulin glycoproteins with a molecular weight not exceeding 1000. They carry only one or two antigenic determinants.

3. True
Haptoglobins bind to free haemoglobin.

4. True
Three types of haptoglobin can be distinguished by the use of electrophoresis. Each type is determined by the interaction of two co-dominant somatic genes Hp^1 and Hp^2.

5. False
Haptoglobins play no part in the rheumatoid factor. The latter is an autoantibody directed against the Gm antigens on the heavy chain of IgG molecules. Gm antigens form allotypes of immunoglobulin molecules. This characteristic of IgG molecules is determined by a dominant autosomal gene.

Section 8. DISORDERS OF THE PLASMA PROTEINS

8.1 The total plasma protein level is low in:

1. patients suffering from protein losing enteropathy
2. patients suffering from cardiac failure associated with oedema
3. oedema due to nephrotic syndrome
4. nutritional oedema
5. patients suffering from chronic liver disease

1. True
Protein losing enteropathy is associated with a massive loss of protein into the gastrointestinal tract. This

186

results in a fall in the plasma proteins and the development of oedema in dependent parts. This syndrome is associated with hypertrophic gastritis and the Zollinger Ellison Syndrome.

2. False
Hypoproteinaemia does not occur or play any part in the oedema associated with cardiac failure. The protein content of the oedema associated with congestive heart failure is that of a typical transudate. The specific gravity is low, the protein content is less than 10 g/l and no fibrinogen is present. The oedema of cardiac failure is partially due to the rise in venous pressure and partially due to an increased vascular permeability caused by the poor blood flow.

3. True
The nephrotic syndrome is associated with a very severe proteinuria, due to an increased glomerular capillary permeability for protein, the loss being chiefly albumin. A fall in plasma protein concentration follows, followed by oedema.

4. True
Nutritional oedema is accompanied by a fall in the plasma protein level which may be reduced to half the normal level. The fall in colloid osmotic pressure is probably the major cause of the generalised oedema seen in this condition although there is seldom any correlation between the absolute value and the severity of the oedema.

5. True
The hepatocytes synthesise all the albumin present in the circulation. Thus in severe cirrhosis in which the number of hepatocytes is decreased and the function of those remaining is reduced hypoproteinaemia develops. This contributes to the development of peripheral oedema by causing a fall in the colloid osmotic pressure but in addition secondary hyperaldosteronism induces sodium retention and aggravates the condition.

8.2 The nephrotic syndrome is associated with:

1. no evidence of sodium retention
2. high levels of aldosterone in the urine
3. high levels of antidiuretic hormone in the urine

4. an increased blood volume
5. hypolipidaemia

1. False
The nephrotic syndrome is accompanied by an increase in aldosterone secretion from the adrenal cortex. This causes sodium retention and oedema, the latter being reduced by a salt free diet.

2. True
As a result of increased secretion of this hormone high levels are found in the urine.

3. True
The secretion of the antidiuretic hormone (ADH) by the posterior pituitary is increased in the nephrotic syndrome in response to the falling blood volume. The result is to increase the absorption of water by the distal tubules. High levels of ADH will be found in the urine.

4. False
The blood volume is diminished in the nephrotic syndrome due to the low plasma protein level which diminishes the colloid osmotic pressure.

5. False
A common feature of the nephrotic syndrome is hyperlipidaemia, the increase in levels of low density lipoproteins often being considerable. This biochemical change is unexplained but it leads to yellow radial streaking of the cortex of the kidney due to deposition of lipids in the tubular epithelial cells and interstitial tissue of the cortex, the lipid being reabsorbed by the tubules from the glomerular filtrate.

8.3 Secondary hypogammaglobulinaemia occurs in:

1. sarcoidosis
2. congestive cardiac failure
3. malnutrition
4. protein losing enteropathy
5. nephrotic syndrome

1. False
Sarcoidosis is accompanied by a depression of cutaneous delayed hypersensitivity reactions including

tuberculin reactivity and the ability to be sensitised with DNCB. There is, however, no evidence of depressed B-lymphocyte function and a secondary hypogammaglobulinaemia does not occur.

2. False
There is no evidence of hypogammaglobulinaemia in association with the oedema of congestive cardiac failure.

3. True
Protein-calorie malnutrition is associated with a functional defect of both the T-lymphocytes and B-lymphocytes. This leads to secondary hypo-gammaglobulinaemia associated with decreased immunoglobulin synthesis.

4. True
This uncommon but serious cause of hypoprotein-aemia is associated with a variety of diseases of the gastrointestinal tract including gastric carcinoma, hypertrophic gastritis, Whipple's disease, Crohn's disease, steatorrhoea and ulcerative colitis.

5. True
Protein loss due to failure of reabsorption from the renal tubules can cause a depression of the serum immunoglobulins as well as albumin.

8.4 A monoclonal gammopathy occurs in the following diseases:

1. Lepromatous leprosy
2. Kala-azar
3. Multiple myeloma
4. Lymphatic leukaemia
5. Active chronic hepatitis

1. and 2. False
In both leprosy and kala-azar a specific defect in T-lymphocyte immunity to the infecting organism is present. The result is a widespread dissemination of the organism throughout the skin, as in lepromatous leprosy, or organs as in systemic leishmaniasis. These forms of disease are associated with negative delayed hypersensitivity tests to antigens from the infecting organisms but B-lymphocyte function is not affected and consequently high levels of antibody

to the infecting organism are present. An associated generalised polyclonal increase in immunoglobulin synthesis also occurs.

3. True
The term monoclonal gammopathy or 'M' protein means that an increase has occurred in a group of immunoglobulins all of which fall within a very narrow electrophoretic range. This is a particular feature of multiple myeloma, a disease due to the malignant proliferation of what is presumably a single clone of plasma cells although monoclonal gammopathies can occur in patients with other conditions. These include malignant disease and even merely increasing age.

4. True
Monoclonal gammopathy may occur in chronic lymphatic leukaemia. One particular form is heavy chain disease in which the M protein is a part of the Fc fragment of the immunoglobulin.

5. False
Active chronic hepatitis is associated with a polyclonal increase in immunoglobulins, anti-nuclear factor, rheumatoid factor and anti-mitochondrial and antismooth muscle auto-antibodies. As well as liver involvement there may be other evidence of immunological disease such as arthritis.

8.5 The following conditions are associated with a polyclonal gammopathy:

1. Waldenström's macroglobulinaemia
2. Rheumatoid arthritis
3. Down's syndrome
4. Wiskott–Aldrich syndrome
5. Cirrhosis of the liver

1. False
Waldenström's macroglobulinaemia is a relatively mild condition compared with multiple myeloma. Clinically this condition is associated with anaemia, lymphadenopathy, splenomegaly and hepatomegaly. However, unlike the IgG, IgA, IgD and IgE myelomas deposits do not develop in the bones. The

reason for the relative mildness of this disease is unknown.

2. True
The term polyclonal gammopathy means that a general rise in immunoglobulins has occurred. This is a feature of a wide range of chronic infections and chronic inflammatory conditions such as tuberculosis, leprosy, systemic leishmaniasis and rheumatoid arthritis. In addition conditions such as systemic lupus erythematosus are also associated with a polyclonal rise in immunoglobulins.

3. False
There is no evidence of increased immunoglobulin synthesis in Down's syndrome which is a genetic defect associated with three instead of the normal pair of number 21 chromosomes.

4. False
The Wiskott–Aldrich syndrome is a condition in which there is atopic eczema, thrombocytopenia and an increased susceptibility to infection in infants. It is a sex linked recessive condition accompanied by a defect in antibody production, low levels of IgM and defective T-cell function.

5. True
A polyclonal rise in circulating immunoglobulins is a feature of hepatic cirrhosis. The cause is unknown.

Section 9. DISORDERS OF CALCIUM METABOLISM

9.1 The normal level of ionised calcium in the plasma is maintained by the following mechanisms:

1. The secretion of calcitonin
2. The presence of 1,25 $(OH)_2$ D_3
3. Parathyroid hormone secretion
4. Renal tubular conservation
5. The circulating level of magnesium

1. True
Calcitonin is a peptide hormone. The stimulus to an increased secretion of this hormone is an increase in

the plasma calcium concentration. An increase in calcitonin lowers the plasma calcium concentration.

2. True
1,25 $(OH)_2$ D_3 is the active metabolite of vitamin D, its major functions are:
  (a) To increase the retention of calcium and phosphate
  (b) To control the mineralisation of bone matrix
In vitamin D deficiency the plasma calcium falls.

3. True
Parathyroid hormone regulates the rate of activation of bone metabolism and maintains the plasma calcium concentration at a sufficient level to ensure the optimum function of a wide variety of cells.

4. True
Approximately 10 000 mg (247 000 mmol) of calcium are filtered through the glomeruli but renal conservation is so complete that only 1 per cent is daily excreted in the urine.

5. False
Changes in the level of circulating magnesium can occur without the serum calcium level altering. However, parathyroid hormone does play some part in the regulation of this ion since hypomagnesaemia may occur in hyperparathyroidism.

9.2 Hypercalcaemia is associated with:

1. increased excitability of the neuromuscular apparatus
2. band keratitis
3. metastatic calcification
4. prolonged Q–T interval
5. renal stones

1. False
Increased excitability of the neuromuscular junction occurs in conditions giving rise to hypocalcaemia, e.g. damage to the parathyroid glands during thyroidectomy. Hypercalcaemia is associated with decreased excitability, about twice as much galvanic current being required to excite a peripheral nerve as in the normal state.

2. True
Band keratitis is particularly common in the hyper-calcaemic state associated with primary hyperpara-thyroidism.

3. True
Metastatic calcification does occur in hypercalcaemia but is not as common in hyperparathyroidism as in hypervitaminosis D.

4. False
The Q–T interval is shortened in any condition giving rise to hypercalcaemia.

5. True
Renal stones, either composed of calcium oxalate or phosphate, occur in hypercalcaemia in association with nephrocalcinosis and hypercalciuria.

9.3 The destruction of bone is associated with the following biochemical changes:

1. An increased secretion of hydroxyproline in the urine
2. An elevated alkaline phosphatase
3. An elevated acid phosphatase
4. An elevated serum calcium
5. Depression of the serum phosphate

1. True
When bone collagen is destroyed most of it is hy-drolysed to its constituent amino acids which are then re-used or degraded further to carbon dioxide and urea. However, 5.8 per cent of collagen is only partially degraded into soluble hydroxyproline-containing peptides which circulate in the blood stream and are excreted in the urine.

2. True
Serum alkaline phosphatase comes from three sites: liver, bone and intestine. In normal subjects liver and bone contribute almost equal amounts and the contribution by the intestinal mucosa is small. In conditions causing bone destruction the alkaline phosphatase rises. However, a similar rise also oc-curs in liver diseases, particularly in biliary cirrhosis. A distinction between liver and bone disease is possible if the concentration of enzymes such as

leucine aminopeptidase which is only produced by the cholangioles is determined.

3. False
This enzyme is synthesised in the prostate and its level is usually elevated in the presence of a malignant prostate particularly if skeletal secondaries are present. Both the alkaline and acid phosphatases may be raised in this situation because typical prostatic secondary deposits are associated not only with destruction but also the laying down of new bone, producing osteoplastic or sclerotic metastases.

4. True
The level of the serum calcium rises in the presence of severe bone destruction, e.g. when generalised osteolytic bone deposits are present leading to hypercalcaemia and metastatic calcification particularly in the kidney.

5. True
The relationship between calcium and phosphate is reciprocal. Any condition, such as bone destruction, which raises the circulating level of calcium is normally associated with a depression of the phosphate concentration.

9.4 Hypercalcaemia and hypercalciuria is caused by:

1. osteolytic secondary deposits in bone
2. hypervitaminosis D, often referred to as vitamin D intoxication
3. parathyroid adenomata or carcinomata.
4. tumours of adrenal medulla
5. primary carcinoma of the kidney.

1. True
All osteolytic secondary deposits cause hypercalcaemia and hypercalciuria because of the breakdown of bone and the liberation of calcium.

2. True
The administration of excessive quantities of vitamin D leads to an increase in calcium absorption from the gut and hence an increase in the blood calcium followed by hypercalciuria. Given in excessive

amounts over a prolonged period this results in nephrocalcinosis.

3. True
Benign or malignant tumours of the parathyroids or simple hyperplasia results in an increase in the concentration of circulating parathyroid hormone. This causes a variety of effects on the cells found in bone including:
  (a) The activation of adenylcyclase in the osteoblasts
  (b) Stimulation of osteoclast division
The net result is increased bone resorption associated with hypercalcaemia and hypercalciuria.

4. False
Tumours of the adrenal medulla secrete noradrenaline and adrenaline which have no effect on the skeleton or the serum calcium.

5. False
The only hormone secreted by the kidney is erythropoietin which is one of the many factors controlling the production of red cells. This hormone is produced by the action of an enzyme-like factor on a plasma substrate. The regulation of the rate at which erythropoietin is produced is determined by the relationship between the oxygen supply to the kidney and the metabolic needs of that organ.

9.5 Excessive osteoid tissue is formed in:

1. vitamin D deficiency
2. Muslim women
3. patients on anticonvulsant drugs
4. patients on long-term anticoagulant therapy
5. long-standing obstructive jaundice

1. True
The metabolites of vitamin D are essential for the absorption of calcium from the gut and in addition they also have a direct action on bone, promoting resorption. How vitamin D promotes bone, mineralisation is not yet fully established but the effect of a vitamin D deficiency is to cause bone which is laid down to be poorly calcified.

195

2. True
Muslim women may have a relatively high incidence of osteomalacia in which excessive osteoid occurs in the skeleton because their extensive clothing prevents vitamin D_3 synthesis from 7-dihydrocholesterol by ultra violet light.

3. True
Several anticonvulsant drugs if given for prolonged periods may lead to the excessive formation of osteoid. This is probably due to the stimulus these drugs give to the production in the liver of isoenzymes which convert vitamin D to inactive metabolites.

4. False
Long term anticoagulant therapy has no effect on vitamin D synthesis or bone development.

5. True
The absorption of vitamin D requires the presence of bile salts, absorption normally occurring in the lower part of the small intestine. The vitamin is then hydroxylated in the liver and altered in the kidney to its biologically most active form. A vitamin D deficiency is, therefore, theoretically possible in long standing obstructive jaundice.

9.6 The sites in which metastatic calcification occurs are:

1. the pyramids of the kidney
2. the wall of the inferior vena cava
3. old tuberculous lesions
4. atheroma
5. the cornea

1. True
This is the commonest site of metastatic calcification and results in nephrocalcinosis. It may occur in hypercalcaemia associated with hypercalciuria regardless of the cause.

2. False
Calcification is rare in the walls of veins, possibly because of the high CO_2 content of venous blood and the low pH.

3. False
The calcification which occurs in old tuberculous lesions is known as dystrophic calcification. It occurs in tuberculous lesions because of the high fat content of caseous pus. This is due to the high lipid content of the *M. tuberculosis* which is liberated from the bacillus when it dies.

4. False
Calcification certainly occurs in atheromatous plaques but this is dystrophic in nature. Calcium is deposited because of the high concentration of lipid in atheroma.

5. True
The cornea is frequently affected and the condition can be discovered during life by slit lamp examination.

9.7 Osteoporosis differs from osteomalacia in that:

1. the radiographic density of the skeleton is reduced in the former and not the latter
2. the remaining bone in the former presents a normal histological appearance
3. major changes occur in the epiphyses in the former
4. pseudofractures are commoner in the former than the latter
5. excess osteoid tissue is present in the former

1. False
This is one of the cardinal changes in both conditions. It is a reflection of the decrease in the amount of calcified bone. In osteomalacia osteoid is laid down which is not calcified and in osteoporosis the bone matrix is diminished in amount thus decreasing overall bone density.

2. True
Osteoporosis is associated with a decrease in the total amount of bone although the cellular composition of the remainder is normal as also is the degree of mineralisation and organisation. The total decrease in bone may be due to decreased formation, increased bone resorption or a combination of both.

3. False

Changes in the epiphyses are characteristic of osteomalacia if its onset occurs before the epiphyses fuse as in rickets. This disease is caused by vitamin D deficiency and is associated with a failure of mineralisation of the osteoid and the cartilage of the epiphyseal growth plate. Radiological examination of affected long bones shows wide, irregular fuzzy, cupped metaphyses, thin bony cortices and the late appearance of epiphyseal centres.

4. False

Pseudofractures are typical of osteomalacia. The radiological picture is one of a linear zone of translucency cutting across at right angles to and usually affecting only one cortex.

5. False

Excess osteoid is the characteristic feature of osteomalacia. Calcification, however, fails to occur in the absence of vitamin D.

9.8 Urinary hydroxyproline excretion may be increased in:

1. Paget's disease of bone
2. Cushing's syndrome
3. hypopituitarism in children
4. hyperthyroidism
5. extensive fractures

The answer is:

1. **True**
2. **False**
3. **False**
4. **True**
5. **True**

When collagen is destroyed it is first degraded into soluble peptides containing the amino acid hydroxyproline. Most of the hydroxyproline is then degraded into carbon dioxide and urea but a small percentage circulates in the plasma to be excreted in the urine. Although the relationship between hydroxyproline excretion and bone resorption is not as simple as first appeared elevated values are normally taken as evidence that such a change is taking place.

In normal circumstances 8 to 10 per cent of the hydroxyproline in the dietary gelatin and collagen appears in the urine and in addition recently synthesised collagen also contributes to the total urinary hydroxyproline.

In Paget's disease, which is a primary disorder of skeletal remodelling, the rapid turnover of bone leads to high urinary levels of hydroxyproline whereas in Cushing's disease attrition of the bone matrix leads to generalised osteoporosis. Weakening of the vertebral bodies produces bulging of the intervertebral discs giving rise to the classical radiological appearance of 'codfish' vertebrae but no rise in the urinary hydroxyproline value occurs because the bone matrix remains normal.

9.9 The following pathological changes can occur in metabolic bone disease:

1. Osteoporosis
2. Localised areas of skeletal involvement
3. Osteomalacia
4. Osteopetrosis
5. Osteitis fibrosa cystica

1. True
Osteoporosis is defined as a decrease in radiographic density of the bone due to loss of the total amount of bone. The remaining bone is, however, normal in terms of its cellular appearance, degree of mineralisation and organisation.

2. False
Albright defined metabolic bone disease as one in which a generalised disorder of bone arises as a consequence of a disturbance in general body metabolism. All bones are, therefore, involved although some may exhibit more pronounced changes than others.

3. True
This change is accompanied histologically by decreased mineralisation and the presence of excess osteoid. Radiologically typical changes occur in the epiphyses as in rickets and in many patients pseudo fractures known as Looser's zones occur. These are

linear zones of translucency, cutting across at right angles to and usually affecting only one cortex.

4. True

Osteopetrosis is associated with an increase in the density of the bone on radiological examination. Histologically the bone is immature and does not undergo normal remodelling.

5. True

Radiological examination of the bone in this condition shows cyst formation and areas of bone erosion. Histologically the affected bone shows marked osteoclastic activity and secondary fibrosis.

Section 10. OEDEMA AND AMYLOID

10.1 Oedema occurs in:

1. Cushing's syndrome
2. primary aldosteronism
3. Zollinger–Ellison syndrome
4. Klinefelter's syndrome
5. pregnancy

1. True

Cushing's syndrome is caused by the excessive production of both mineralo- and gluco-corticoids by the adrenal cortex, due either to the presence of hyperplasia, an adenoma or carcinoma. Sodium retention follows with the result that oedema develops. Additional factors are the associated hypertension and a change in the chemical structure of the interstitial tissue allowing more fluid retention.

2. False

Primary aldosteronism, which is most frequently caused by an adrenal cortical adenoma, is associated with sodium and water retention which causes hypertension but oedema does not occur possibly because increasing amounts of sodium ion are excreted by the kidneys.

3. True

The Zollinger–Ellison syndrome which is caused by a non-β cell tumour of the pancreatic islet cells known as a gastrinoma causes a protein losing enteropathy due to the effect of the excessive amounts of acid which are secreted. This causes an enteritis, the result of which is the loss of large amounts of protein into the gut followed by generalised oedema.

4. False
This syndrome is not associated with oedema. It is one of the commonest chromosomal disorders resulting from the presence of a Y chromosome together with a second X, the Y chromosome ensures the formation of the testes and masculine development but the second X prevents the development of the testes.

5. True
Pregnancy is associated with fluid retention which thus gives rise to oedema particularly in the dependent parts. In late pregnancy hypertension and pre-eclampsia may lead to worsening of the condition.

10.2 Angioneurotic oedema which is a neurovascular event is associated with:

1. depression
2. complement deficiency
3. immunoglobulin E
4. menstruation
5. Lawrence's transfer factor

1. False
Although the term 'angioneurotic' may suggest an underlying psychiatric disorder this is not so. The term is used to describe an oedema, mainly of the urticarial type which is frequently seen on the face and neck.

2. True
The absence of C1 esterase inhibitor is the cause of hereditary angioneurotic oedema. Affected individuals develop acute attacks of oedematous swelling of the skin which does not pit on pressure or itch. In addition laryngeal oedema may give rise to asphyxia.

3. True
The urticarial attacks associated with angioneurotic oedema are mostly anaphylactoid reactions involv-

ing IgE and are due to the release of vasoactive amines from mast cells as well as activation of the kinin system by kallikrein.

4. False
The salt and water retention associated with the premenstrual period are normally not associated with increased capillary permeability and oedema.

5. False
Lawrence's transfer factor is related to cell-mediated immunity and delayed hypersensitivity reactions in man. Described in 1948 by Lawrence who reported that cell-free extracts of human leucocytes could transfer cell-mediated immunity to non-immunised recipients.

10.3 Pulmonary oedema may occur in patients suffering from:

1. head injuries
2. plague
3. right-sided heart failure
4. hypoproteinaemia
5. nematode infections

1. True
Pulmonary oedema may occur in patients suffering from head injuries, particularly those involving the hind brain. One explanation of this is the association between hind brain injuries and the secretion of massive amounts of adrenaline, the latter causing marked peripheral vasoconstriction. In experimental animals vagotomy prior to the infliction of the head injury inhibits the development of oedema.

2. True
The pulmonary oedema seen in plague victims is chiefly a product of the associated bronchopneumonia and it occurs with extreme rapidity in patients suffering from pneumonic as opposed to the bubonic form of plague. However, pulmonary oedema is a feature of the septicaemia associated with a wide range of micro-organisms.

3. False
Pulmonary oedema occurs in left-sided heart failure and is, therefore, most commonly seen in patients

who have a failing heart due to hypertension, or acute failure due to a myocardial infarct. In the former condition the oedema frequently develops at night when the patient is lying down causing attacks of nocturnal dyspnoea (cardiac asthma), probably because of the increased venous return and perhaps because of the reabsorption of oedema fluid from the legs when recumbent.

4. False
Hypoproteinaemia does not specifically cause pulmonary oedema except as a terminal event when cardiac failure occurs. However, hypoproteinaemia is associated with peripheral dependent oedema.

5. False
Nematode larvae of ankylostomes and ascaris may migrate through the lungs and cause pulmonary eosinophilia. This may be associated with pneumonic consolidation but there is no evidence that they cause pulmonary oedema.

10.4 Amyloid is deposited most frequently in:

1. liver
2. brain
3. spleen
4. lungs
5. kidneys

1. True
Amyloid, which produces a waxy refractile appearance on the cut surface of an affected organ, is deposited in the liver chiefly in the sinusoids of the intermediate zones of the lobules. As the process becomes increasingly extensive marked atrophy of the liver cells occurs but even at an advanced stage liver function is not usually severely impaired.

2. False
The central nervous system is not normally affected in amyloidosis although it may occur in the centre of the degenerative plaques in Alzheimer's dementia, this term being applied to a dementia beginning before the age of 60.

3. True
Amyloid deposits in the spleen take two forms. In

one the Malpighian bodies are changed into trans-
lucent globules by amyloid deposition in their reticulum, hence the term sago spleen, in which
splenomegaly is not marked. In the other form the
change affects the reticulum of the red pulp, the
walls of the venous sinuses and many of the small
arteries. In this latter type the spleen may be palpable and weigh up to 1 kg, this is a rarer condition
than the sago spleen and is only common in tertiary
syphilis.

4. False
The lungs are an infrequent site of amyloid deposition although deposits may occur in primary amyloidosis, i.e. amyloidosis occurring in the absence of
any predisposing cause.

5. True
Renal amyloidosis is particularly important because
once established renal failure is almost inevitable.
The amyloid is deposited upon the basement membranes of the tubules, in the walls of arterioles and
venules and most importantly, in the basement
membrane of the glomerular capillaries. The latter
leads to the capillaries becoming permeable to albumin with the result that heavy proteinuria develops
followed by the nephrotic syndrome.

**10.5 The following conditions are particularly
associated with the deposition of amyloid:**

1. Gas gangrene
2. Leprosy
3. Osteomyelitis
4. Bronchiectasis
5. Pneumococcal pneumonia

1. False
Secondary amyloidosis is a feature of chronic rather
than acute infection.

2. True
Secondary amyloidosis is a frequent cause of death
in lepromatous leprosy, resulting from the renal
failure caused by the renal deposition of amyloid. In
contrast amyloidosis is not a particular feature of
tuberculoid leprosy.

3. True
Secondary amyloid deposits occur in chronic pyogenic osteomyelitis. It is not, however, a particular feature of acute osteomyelitis.

4. True
Bronchiectasis which was usually a sequel of childhood bronchiolitis and bronchopneumonia associated with partial collapse and imperfect resolution was in the past the commonest cause of secondary amyloidosis.

5. False
Acute pneumococcal pulmonary infections do not lead to amyloidosis.

10.6 Secondary amyloidosis occurs in the following conditions:

1. Familial Mediterranean fever
2. Thalassaemia
3. Sickle-cell disease
4. Multiple myeloma
5. Rheumatoid arthritis

1. True
This condition, principally found in people of Mediterranean origin, in inherited as an autosomal recessive trait. Clinically it is characterised by recurring joint and abdominal pains and fever, frequently commencing in childhood. Amyloid deposits develop in the kidneys leading to proteinuria and finally renal failure. Death normally occurs about 10 years after the onset of symptoms.

2. False
This is a haemoglobinopathy occurring chiefly in the Mediterranean region. Amyloidosis does not develop but the condition is complicated by the occurrence of haemosiderosis and cirrhosis of the liver.

3. False
Sickle cell disease is another haemoglobinopathy in which a chronic anaemia develops. The complications of the condition include ulceration of the legs, respiratory infection, cardiomyopathy and thrombotic crises.

4. True

In multiple myeloma deposits of amyloid material may occur in atypical sites such as the heart. There is, therefore, some similarity between this condition and primary amyloidosis in which there is no predisposing cause.

5. True

Rheumatoid arthritis has now replaced chronic pyogenic infection as the commonest cause of secondary amyloidosis. Postmortem examination reveals amyloid deposits in 20 per cent of all cases. This disease is of unknown aetiology but with many immunological features including circulating IgM anti-immunoglobulin antibodies (the rheumatoid factor).

10.7 The essential constituents of amyloid include:

1. immunoglobulins
2. complement
3. albumin
4. starch
5. fibrils

1. True

In primary amyloidosis or amyloidosis associated with multiple myeloma, the major protein which forms the amyloid fibrils has a structure similar to immunoglobulin $\varkappa$ or λ light chains. In hereditary amyloid disease and rheumatoid arthritis the major amyloid protein is not recognised as part of the immunoglobulin molecule.

2. False

The complement proteins are not major components of amyloid although they may occur in low concentrations.

3. False

Albumin is not a major component of amyloid.

4. False

The term amyloid was first used by Rokitansky in 1842, because it stained violet with iodine and sulphuric acid in the same way as starch.

5. True

Amyloid formed in response to prolonged antigenic

stimulation, e.g. following chronic infection, in hereditary amyloidosis and rheumatoid arthritis is chiefly composed of a fibrous protein which forms the amyloid fibrils. This has been termed protein A. An antigenically related protein, SAA, may be found in the serum.

10.8 Amyloidosis may be associated with elevated levels of the following serum proteins:

1. β-lipoprotein
2. SAA
3. IgD
4. M-protein
5. β-microglobulin

1. False
Amyloidosis is not associated with elevated serum levels of β-lipoprotein. An elevation of these components occurs in a number of familial conditions and may lead to atherosclerosis with its attendant complications.

2. True
Amyloid protein A levels are raised in hereditary amyloidosis and in a number of acute and chronic inflammatory conditions which give rise to secondary amyloidosis, including rheumatoid arthritis. A similar elevation occurs in multiple myeloma and the lymphomas.

3. False
IgD is present in low concentration in the serum. Increased levels of IgD may occur in chronic infections or in IgD myelomas.

4. True
The term M-protein is used for the monoclonal immunoglobulin found in a monoclonal gammopathy. Monoclonal gammopathy is one of the features of multiple myeloma which may be associated with a primary amyloid type condition.

5. False
β-microglobulin is protein resembling IgG. It is integrated into the cell membrane together with a glycoprotein to form the HLA human transplantation

antigen although β-microglobulin itself does not carry transplantation antigen specificity.

10.9 Amyloid reacts with the following stains:

1. Thioflavine-T
2. Fluoroscein isothiocyanate
3. Methyl violet
4. Methyl green
5. Congo red

1. True
Thioflavine-T is a fluorochrome which reacts with amyloid. It is particularly useful for demonstrating small glomerular deposits.

2. False
Fluoroscein isothiocyanate does not stain amyloid deposits. It is used to conjugate with antibody in the fluorescent antibody technique.

3. True
Methyl violet is a metachromatic stain, staining normal tissue violet and amyloid pink.

4. False
Methyl green does not stain amyloid deposits. It reacts specifically with DNA and is used as part of the methyl green-pyronin stain (Unna-Pappenheim) which is specific for DNA and RNA.

5. True
The congo red test for amyloid depends on the specificity of this dye for amyloid. Intravenously administered congo red disappears rapidly from the circulation in amyloid disease due to its rapid conjugation with this material. Amyloid material stained with congo red can be seen to best advantage when the tissue is examined in polarised light when a green birefringence can be seen. Biopsy material to establish the presence of amyloid is usually taken from the rectum, gums or kidney.

Section 11. PIGMENTATION

11.1 Generalised pigmentation of the skin occurs in:

1. carcinoma of the head of the pancreas
2. idiopathic haemochromatosis

3. argyria
4. arsenic poisoning
5. black liver disease

1. True
One of the first clinical manifestations of carcinoma of the head of the pancreas may be the onset of jaundice due to increasing compression of the common bile duct. The colour of the skin tends to be olive green due to the retention of biliverdin. Removal of the obstruction does not result in an abrupt return to normal due to the strong affinity of elastic tissue for bile pigments.

2. True
In idiopathic haemochromatosis the excessive absorption of dietary iron causes the total iron content of the body gradually to increase. By middle age the total iron content is four or five times greater than normal. The skin in this disease appears leaden due to the deposition of iron around the sweat glands. In addition excess melanin production also increases the skin pigmentation leading to the alternative name for this condition of Bronze Diabetes.

3. True
The prolonged administration of remedies containing silver preparations is followed by the deposition of brownish granules of silver compounds in the skin, gut wall and basement membrane of the glomeruli and renal collecting tubules.

4. False
Chronic arsenic poisoning leads to arsenical keratosis in which epithelial atrophy, dysplasia, hyperkeratosis and parakeratosis occur.

5. False
This is a synergistic infection found in sheep in which *Cl. oedematiens* is frequently harboured in the liver in the absence of disease. Should the animal become infected with the liver fluke, *Fasciola hepatica*, the local conditions created favour the growth of the clostridia and the animal develops a condition known as black liver disease.

11.2 Patchy skin pigmentation occurs in the following conditions:

1. Peutz–Jegher syndrome

2. Familial polyposis
3. Addison's disease
4. Purpura
5. Vitiligo

1. True
This is a hereditary disorder transmitted as a Mendelian dominant of high penetrance. It is associated with multiple polyps of the small bowel. These lead to recurrent intussusception, and recurrent attacks of abdominal pain together with an iron deficiency anaemia due to blood loss. The external marker of this condition is patchy circumoral melanotic pigmentation together with similar pigmentation of the oral mucosa.

2. False
Pigmentation does not occur in familial polyposis. In the related condition of Gardner's syndrome colonic polyps occur in association with sebaceous cysts, osteomata of the face and skull, desmoid tumours and multiple fibromata.

3. False
Addison's disease is associated with a generalised increase in melanotic pigmentation of the skin due to the excessive release of MSH (melanocyte stimulating hormone) by the hypophysis following the decline of adrenal inhibition.

4. True
Any cause of purpura or bruising leads to temporary localised staining of the skin. This is due to the dermal macrophages retaining some of the iron released from the red cells and incrustation of the collagen molecules with iron.

5. False
Vitiligo is a patchy depigmentation of the skin in which the dendritic cells are abnormal in structure and have lost their ability to oxidase dopa to pigment.

11.3 The following endocrine abnormalities lead to generalised pigmentation:

1. Cushing's disease
2. Carcinoid tumours

3. Zollinger Ellison syndrome
4. Addison's disease
5. Sheehan's syndrome

1. True
Cushing's disease is associated with high plasma ACTH levels. This hormone possesses melanocyte stimulating properties although it is not as potent as MSH.

2. False
Although the face and upper chest may be cyanotic in colour and bright red flushes occur in this syndrome there is no true pigmentation. The flushes are provoked by alcohol and may be inhibited by α-adrenergic blocking agents.

3. False
This syndrome in which a gastrin secreting tumour of the pancreatic islet cells occurs is not associated with pigmentation. A common presenting syndrome is intractable duodenal ulceration.

4. True
Addison's disease follows destruction of the adrenal glands. This leads to very high outputs of ACTH and MSH leading to melanin deposition and striking hyperpigmentation. The agent responsible is believed to be beta-MSH which is an extremely potent pigmentary hormone. The plasma concentration of this hormone is roughly parallel to the degree of hyperpigmentation.

5. False
The appearance of the skin in this condition often provides the first clue to the presence of this condition. A waxy character of the skin, often with myxoedema, is highly suggestive. Melanin pigmentation usually decreases and even the areolae of the breast may become depigmented. These changes help to distinguish Sheehan's syndrome from Addison's disease.

11.4 Idiopathic haemachromotosis is associated with:

1. an excessive production of melanin
2. decreased absorption of iron from the gut

211

3. the deposition of haemosiderin in the liver
4. diabetes
5. females

1. True
Excessive melanin production, cause unknown, does occur in this condition. The generalised pigmentation which occurs has led to the alternative name of Bronze Diabetes. An additional cause of skin pigmentation in this disease is the deposition of iron around the sweat glands.

2. False
The basic fault in idiopathic haemochromatosis is an excessive absorption of dietary iron. This leads to a gradual increase in the body's iron stores which rise from a normal value of 3 to 4 g to amounts in excess of 20 g by middle age.

3. True
Haemosiderin is deposited in the hepatocytes. This leads to their destruction and to the eventual development of cirrhosis.

4. True
Iron is deposited in the parenchymal cells of the pancreas and diabetes eventually develops. It is assumed that the diabetes follows the excessive deposition of iron in the β-cells.

5. False
Haemochromatosis is thirteen times as common in males than females because the latter lose much of the extra iron they absorb by menstruation.

11.5 Haemosiderosis differs from haemochromatosis in that:

1. the former is more common in the Bantu
2. the latter is due to the excessive absorption of iron and the former to excessive dietary intake
3. in the former the excessive iron is mainly deposited in the parenchymal cells whereas in the latter the excess iron is deposited mainly in the macrophages of the liver, spleen and bone marrow
4. in the former cirrhosis does not develop

5. in the latter the level of plasma transferrin is abnormally high.

1. True
The high incidence of haemosiderosis in the Bantu is probably caused by excess dietary iron. This is believed to be due to the large quantities of Kaffir beer, brewed in iron containers, which is consumed by the Bantu.

2. False
The converse is correct. An excessive intake of iron leads to haemosiderosis. Idiopathic haemochromatosis is the result of excessive absorption, the intake being normal.

3. False
The converse is correct thus explaining the high incidence of diabetes and cirrhosis in the latter condition.

4. True
In haemosiderosis iron is found in the liver but it is deposited in the macrophages and not in the parenchymal cells and, therefore, cirrhosis does not occur.

5. False
The plasma transferrin is normal in quantity and not qualitatively abnormal in either condition.

Section 12. DISEASES OF THE LIVER AND GALL BLADDER

12.1 Obstruction of the common bile duct is associated with the following biochemical abnormalities:

1. A greater increase in the serum concentration of bilirubin diglucuronide than bilirubin monoglucuronide
2. An increase in the serum concentration of unconjugated bilirubin
3. A decrease in the faecal stercobilinogen content
4. An increase in faecal fat
5. An increase in urinary urobilinogen

1. False
The concentration of bilirubin monoglucuronide is increased relative to that of diglucuronide because biliary tract obstruction is associated with an impairment of conjugation as well as the more obvious obstructive element.

2. False
The serum concentration of conjugated bilirubin rises. Conjugated pigment is attached to serum protein, mainly albumin.

3. True
The stercobilinogen content of the faeces is dependent upon the amount of bilirubin excreted into the bowel. This is then converted to stercobilinogen by the intestinal flora.

4. True
The fat content of the faeces increases because in the absence of bile salts in the bowel fat absorption is diminished.

5. False
The urinary urobilinogen must decrease because it is derived from the stercobilinogen absorbed from the gastrointestinal tract some of which is excreted by the kidneys.

12.2 Haemolytic jaundice is associated with:

1. an increase in the concentration of bilirubin diglucuronide in the bile
2. the presence of bilirubin in the urine
3. an increase in the serum alkaline phosphatase
4. a decrease in unconjugated bilirubin in the serum
5. an increase in urobilinogen in the urine

1. True
Increased amounts of unconjugated bilirubin are presented to the liver cell, because the liver cells are normal. Conjugation proceeds normally and increased quantities of the diglucuronide appear in the bile.

2. False
Unconjugated bilirubin is insoluble in water unlike the conjugated forms and, therefore, does not appear in the urine in haemolytic anaemia, hence the term, acholuric jaundice.

3. False
The serum alkaline phosphatase concentration increases in obstructive and hepatocellular jaundice. Its concentration does not rise in haemolytic jaundice unless haemolysis has been associated with the formation of pigment stones which have then caused obstruction of the common bile duct.

4. False
In haemolytic disease, an increase in bilirubin occurs, principally of the unconjugated fraction. The total bilirubin rarely exceeds 5 mg/dl (85 μmol/l) because the rate of excretion increases as the total bilirubin rises and a plateau is quickly reached. Greater values suggest concomitant hepatic parenchymal disease.

5. True
Because increased quantities of conjugated bilirubin are being excreted into the gastrointestinal tract greater quantities of stercobilininogen are formed, absorbed and then excreted by the kidney as urobilinogen which is then converted to urobilin.

12.3 The common causes of cirrhosis of the liver in Great Britain are:

1. alcohol
2. various drugs such as halothane and paracetamol
3. active chronic hepatitis
4. haemochromatosis
5. cryptogenic

1. True
In all series published in Great Britain alcohol is the second commonest cause of cirrhosis of the liver. The incidence of cirrhosis in alcoholics is around 1:10 but there is no clear explanation why some alcoholics develop cirrhosis and others remain immune. However, the frequency of cirrhosis increases with the duration of the abuse and the greater the quantity of alcohol consumed.

2. False
A large number of drugs may damage the liver. Predictable damage follows the inhalation of carbon tetrachloride whereas other drugs such as mono-

215

amine oxidase inhibitors of the hydrazine group, e.g. phenelzine, may or may not produce hepatic damage. Three factors appear to be important in the latter group, these include:

(a) genetic differences in the rate of drug metabolism
(b) quantitative differences in drug metabolism
(c) immunological mechanisms

3. True
Although the incidence of cirrhosis in active chronic hepatitis varies according to the particular survey examined in some this cause of chronic liver disease accounts for approximately a quarter of all cases.

4. False
Although haemochromatosis causes cirrhosis it is a relatively rare cause in Britain.

5. True
Cryptogenic cirrhosis in which the cause is unknown is the commonest of all causes of cirrhosis in Great Britain.

It should be appreciated that outside Great Britain other causes of cirrhosis assume a greater importance. Thus in the USA alcoholic cirrhosis is commoner and in countries in which schistosomiasis is commonplace this produces a form of liver disease in which the chief histological picture is one of extensive fibrosis.

12.4 In liver failure the following biochemical abnormalities may be found:

1. A decrease in the plasma albumin concentration
2. An increase in the plasma globulin
3. An increase in the blood ammonium concentration
4. A rise in the blood urea
5. Impaired glucose tolerance

1. True
The plasma albumin concentration usually falls in chronic liver disease, the majority of patients with cirrhosis having low albumin synthesis rates and small albumin pools.

2. True
The plasma globulin level is frequently increased in patients with cirrhosis because bacterial antigens derived from the gut may have access to the systemic circulation especially if a porta-caval shunt has been performed. In patients with auto-immune liver disease as part of the primary disease process serum autoantibodies will be present.

3. True
Ammonium is produced by the deamination of aminoacids and other nitrogenous substances in muscle, brain, kidney and the colon and cannot be converted to urea by the failing liver.

4. False
The blood urea does not rise unless there is associated renal failure because the ammonium cannot be converted into urea (see above).

5. True
Glucose tolerance is impaired in patients with acute hepatitis and reverts to normal with their clinical recovery. In fulminating hepatic failure the initial changes are similar and hypoglycaemia may supervene.

12.5 A diminution in the bile salt pool and hence a diminished concentration of bile salts in the bile occurs:

1. in jejunal diverticulosis
2. in diseases affecting the terminal ileum such as Crohn's disease
3. due to the eating of refined carbohydrates
4. in ulcerative colitis
5. in congenital deficiency of cholesterol 7α-hydroxylase

1. False
Bile salt depletion does not occur in jejunal diverticulosis because the absorption of bile salts occurs in the terminal ileum.

2. True
Bile salts are absorbed in the terminal ileum. Reabsorption is essential to preserve the enterohepatic circulation of the bile salts. If the terminal ileum is

destroyed by disease or it is resected a diminished bile salt pool inevitably occurs. Because an adequate concentration of bile salts is required to hold the cholesterol in micelles any condition lowering the concentration of bile salts leads to an increased incidence of cholesterol gall stones.

3. True
There is some animal evidence that an acquired deficiency of the enzyme, cholesterol 7α-hydroxylase, follows the eating of refined carbohydrate. Deficiency of this enzyme causes a reduction in bile salt formation.

4. False
The diarrhoea associated with ulcerative colitis has no effect on the bile salt pool since the absorption of bile salts has already taken place in the terminal ileum.

5. True
A congenital deficiency of this enzyme leads to failure of bile salt synthesis.

12.6 Excessive cholesterol is excreted by the hepatocytes:

1. when the diet contains excessive amounts of polyunsaturated fatty acids
2. in response to excessive secretion of testosterone
3. when an individual is excessively obese
4. when anticoagulants are administered in large doses
5. when calorie intake is diminished

1. True
Both a diet containing an excess of polyunsaturated fatty acids and the administration of drugs such as Clofibrate increase the output of cholesterol.

2. False
Oestrogens increase cholesterol excretion. This is believed to be one of the causes of the greater incidence of 'metabolic stones' (cholesterol stones), in women.

3. True
Excessive obesity, probably because of the increase of body fat, causes an increase in the synthesis and excretion of cholesterol by the liver cells.

4. False
Anticoagulants have no effect on cholesterol metabolism.

5. False
A short-term increase in calorie intake may be associated with an increase in cholesterol excretion.

12.7 The main constituents of gall stones are:

1. calcium sulphate
2. cholesterol
3. calcium palmitate
4. calcium bilirubinate
5. amorphous materials

1. False
No calcium sulphate is excreted in the bile but one third of the crystalline matter in stones found in Great Britain is calcium carbonate.

2. True
Cholesterol is the main constituent of gall stones in the developed countries. Supersaturation of the fasting gall bladder bile with cholesterol, associated with the possibility of precipitation, occurs in the presence of an alteration in the concentration of the twin solubilisers of cholesterol, bile salts and lecithin.

3. True
Calcium palmitate is one of the lesser components of gall stones.

4. True
Calcium bilirubinate is the major pigment found in pigment stones.

5. True
The amorphous material found in pigment stones is important because 90 per cent of such stones is composed of this as yet unidentified material.

12.8 Gall stones are associated with the following diseases:

1. Viral hepatitis
2. Cirrhosis of the liver

3. Haemolytic jaundice
4. Obesity
5. Raised serum triglycerides

1. False
Liver damage associated with viral hepatitis causes no increase in the incidence of gall stones.

2. False
Cirrhosis, although associated in the end stage with severe liver damage, does not increase the incidence of gall stones.

3. True
Any form of haemolytic jaundice which is sufficiently severe to cause an increase in the bilirubin content of the bile may be associated with the development of pigment stones. The classical example of this is congenital spherocytosis.

4. True
In one study of the incidence of gall stones in women below the age of fifty those with gall stones were 10 kilograms heavier than those without.

5. True
The incidence of gall stones is increased in conditions leading to a hyperlipidaemia causing an excess of serum triglycerides but not hypercholesterolaemia.

12.9 Severe liver failure is associated with:

1. mucosal bleeding
2. encephalopathy
3. bronchopneumonia
4. venous thrombosis
5. decreased resistance to infection

1. True
Mucosal bleeding from the upper gastrointestinal tract is relatively common and accounts for death in approximately 20 per cent of all cases of advanced liver failure. Bleeding occurs from mucosal erosions and can be prevented by the administration of H_2 receptor antagonists.

2. True
The encephalopathy associated with severe liver failure is believed to be due to the presence in the circulation of many low and middle molecular weight toxins. Among the former some are water soluble such as ammonium and aminoacids and others such as the phenolic acids, fatty acids, bile acids and bilirubin are bound to the plasma proteins.

3. True
Pulmonary complications in the form of bronchopneumonia are very common in severe liver failure due to the depression of the respiratory centre and a decreased resistance to infection.

4. False
Thrombosis is uncommon in severe liver disease because the synthesis of clotting factors is diminished.

5. True
The susceptibility to infection is increased in severe liver disease because the circulating toxins depress polymorphonuclear leucocyte activity and complement deficiency impairs bacterial opsonisation.

12.10 The following biochemical disturbances occur in fulminating hepatic failure:

1. Metabolic acidosis
2. Hyperkalaemia
3. Hypoglycaemia
4. Fall in pO_2
5. Hypernatraemia

1. False
In the early stages of coma a prominent feature is hyperventilation leading to a respiratory alkalosis.

2. False
In about 50 per cent hypokalaemia occurs. This is partly due to haemodilution because the renal excretion of water is diminished.

3. True
A rapid fall in the blood sugar occurs and may lead to irreversible brain damage.

4. True
The respiratory centre is depressed leading to decreased respiration. In addition pulmonary oedema, infection and intrapulmonary shunting occurs.

5. False
Hyponatraemia rather than hypernatraemia occurs because of the retention of water.

12.11 The following coagulation factors are generated in the liver:

1. Factor II
2. Factor IV
3. Factor VI
4. Factor XI
5. Factor X

The liver generates coagulation factors II, V, VII, IX and X and all except Factor V are vitamin K dependent. Deficiencies of these factors together with disturbances in fibrinogen metabolism and thrombocytopenia account for the bleeding diathesis that accompanies both acute and chronic liver disease.

The correct answer to this question is, therefore,
1. True
2. False
3. False
4. True
5. True

Section 13. CARCINOGENESIS

13.1 A hereditary predisposition to the development of tumours occurs at the following sites:

1. Retina
2. Colon
3. Lung
4. Skin
5. Stomach

1. True
Approximately 6 per cent of all cases of retinoblastoma are familial, genetic transmission being due to

an autosomal dominant gene of poor penetrance. Some patients also suffer from mental deficiency and other tumours such as osteosarcomas. Approximately one half of the familial cases are bilateral.

2. True
The colonic disorder associated with malignancy which is commonly transmitted as an autosomal dominant is polyposis coli. This condition can be transmitted by either sex and in some families the responsible gene is recessive with poor penetrance. The onset of malignant disease in the form of multiple adenocarcinomas of the colon and rectum is preceded by the appearance of hundreds of adenomatous polyps which become evident during puberty, malignancy developing some fifteen years later.

3. False
No inherited tumours of the lung have been described although there may be an inherited predisposition to the development of tumours in conditions in which external stimuli, such as smoking, are at work. This hypothesis remains, however, unconfirmed.

4. True
A variety of skin tumours, included among which are malignant melanomas and certain basal cell carcinoma of early childhood, show a hereditary predisposition. In addition xeroderma pigmentosum, which is associated with the development of basal and squamous cell carcinomas, is inherited in the manner of an autosomal recessive disease.

5. False
Carcinoma of the stomach shows no particular hereditary predisposition although this tumour is commoner in individuals possessing blood group A.

13.2 Recognised precancerous conditions include:

1. the intestinal polyps of the small bowel occurring in the Peutz–Jegher syndrome
2. the colonic polyps of familial polyposis
3. xeroderma pigmentosum
4. Bowen's disease
5. Molluscum sebaceum

1. False

The polyps of the small intestine in this hereditary disease, which is transmitted as a Mendelian dominant of high penetrance, are highly differentiated. They are better regarded as hamartomata than true tumours. Rare cases associated with malignant degeneration have been reported.

2. True

The polyps of familial polyposis first make their appearance in affected siblings in early adolescence. They become progressively more numerous, particularly in the distal end of the large bowel and finally become malignant in the early thirties.

3. True

Xeroderma pigmentosum is associated with a genetically determined absence of an enzyme which in the normal individual excises pyrimidine bases of DNA which have become irreversibly coupled by ultra violet rays allowing their replacement by normal bases. The disturbance of nucleic acid metabolism causes an increased frequency of mutations some of which lead to the early development of malignancy.

4. True

Bowen's disease commonly arises in non-exposed areas of the skin forming rounded reddish patches which slowly spread. The epidermis shows marked hyperplasia in which cellular de-differentiation is common. This disease is a form of carcinoma *in situ* from which invasion eventually occurs.

5. False

This tumour-like lesion occurs predominantly on the face and has a natural history of approximately six months. A nodule appears which grows rapidly for about eight weeks during which time the histological picture resembles that of a squamous carcinoma. After this the lesion stabilises and the exuberant epithelium which has formed slowly keratinises. This is then discharged and the lesion heals.

13.3 The following pathological conditions can be regarded as precancerous:

1. Paget's disease of bone
2. Leukoplakia

3. Fibroadenosis of the breast
4. Duodenal ulceration
5. Cervical erosions

1. True
Paget's disease of bone is a chronic bone dystrophy of unknown aertiology chiefly affecting the vertebrae, skull and pelvis. Affected bones become thickened and more vascular. Although not considered to be a metabolic defect the serum alkaline phosphatase is raised, a finding which indicates an increase in osteoblastic activity. Osteosarcoma, fibrosarcoma and chondrosarcoma develop in about 10 per cent of all cases.

2. True
Leukoplakia is a clinical term indicating the presence of white patches in a squamous epithelial mucous membrane. The condition affects the oral cavity and the vulva. In the mouth the condition is believed to be precipitated by chronic irritation. The whiteness of the affected epithelial surface is due to thickening of the epithelium and prolongation of the rete pegs. The papillae contain a chronic inflammatory infiltrate. As time passes the whiteness of the epithelium is converted to reddening due to a loss of cellular thickness and finally a carcinoma *in situ* develops leading eventually to invasive squamous carcinoma.

3. False
Fibroadenosis of the breast, previously known as chronic mastitis and now as generalised cystic mastopathy, does not predispose to neoplastic change unless it is accompanied by marked epithelial hyperplasia. The latter is one of the four possible pathological changes seen in the breast, the others being fibrosis, cyst formation and adenosis. Adenosis indicates the formation of new breast lobules and/or the enlargement of pre-existing ones. The epithelial hyperplasia is referred to as epitheliosis, a term coined by Dawson to indicate hyperplasia of the ductal and acinar epithelium. It is only when this change is marked that the condition can be regarded as precancerous.

4. False
Neoplastic changes do not appear to supervene in

225

duodenal ulceration. This must be compared with the situation in gastric ulceration in which approximately 5 per cent of simple ulcers eventually become malignant.

5. False
The term cervical erosion is applied to the appearance of a red area around the external os spreading onto the exocervix. Histological examination shows that the normal opaque squamous epithelium has been replaced by transparent columnar epithelium. Should the replacement involve the cervical glands an appearance may be produced which is sometimes mistakenly interpreted as early invasive carcinomatous change.

13.4 The following are carcinogenic:

1. Infra-red radiation
2. Ultra-violet radiation
3. House dust
4. Soot
5. Moulds

1. False
Long wave infra-red irradiation is not associated with tumour development.

2. True
Ultra-violet light is a potent carcinogenic agent particularly in fair individuals. In Australia and South Africa, areas in which there is considerable exposure to UVR, individuals working out of doors may first develop actinic keratoses which later become squamous or basal cell skin cancers.

3. False
There are no carcinogens in normal house dust. This should be compared to some industrial occupations, e.g. workers in asbestos factories, in which dust may play an important role in the development of malignant disease. A condition associated with house dust is allergy, causing hay fever and bronchial asthma, chiefly due to antigens from the house dust mite, *Dermatophagoides pteronyssinus*.

4. True
Soot is a carcinogenic agent because of its contained

coal tar products including 3.4 benzpyrene. Cancer of the scrotum occurring in chimney sweeps was the first of the occupational cancers to be described by Percival Pott in 1775.

5. True
Aflatoxin derived from the mould *Aspergillus flavus* is a particular contaminant of ground nut meal and may cause liver cancer in man.

13.5 The following chemicals are carcinogens:

1. 3.4 benzpyrene
2. 2.4 dinitrofluorobenzene
3. β-naphthylamine
4. Acetyl salicyclic acid
5. 4-dimethylamino-azobenzene

1. True
3.4 benzpyrene is the most important carcinogen in coal tar. Applied to the skin squamous cell cancer develops and when subcutaneously injected in experimental animals it will produce sarcomas. The inhalation of fumes containing 3.4 benzpyrene could be a cause of bronchial carcinoma.

2. False
DNFB is a potent contact sensitiser, but has not as yet been found to be carcinogenic in man or in experimental animals.

3. True
β-naphthylamine is a constituent of an antioxidant once used in the rubber industry. Individuals working in contact with this substance were found to develop carcinoma of the bladder. Similar tumours can be produced in dogs fed on β-naphthylamine.

4. False
Aspirin is a potent cause of gastric erosions and haemorrhages, but so far no association has been found between it and tumour formation.

5. True
4-dimethylamino-azobenzene or butter yellow has been used for colouring foodstuffs, fed to rats and mice it is a potent inducer of hepatic cancers.

13.6 The following occupations have been or remain associated with a high incidence of cancer:

1. Coal mining
2. Nickel workers
3. Asbestos workers
4. Dye industry
5. Tobacco industry

1. False
Although there is a high incidence of pneumoconiosis, silicosis, tuberculosis and chronic bronchitis in coal miners, there is no evidence of an increased incidence of neoplasia directly related to this industry. Coal tar on the other hand contains potent carcinogens.

2. True
A higher incidence of bronchial cancer and cancer of the nasal sinuses occurs in workers in contact with nickel or chrome. This is related to the inhalation of dust containing these materials.

3. True
Workers who inhale asbestos have a higher than normal incidence of all types of cancer of the lung. The inhalation of blue asbestos is particularly associated with the development of mesotheliomas.

4. True
Aniline dyes such as α-naphthylamine, β-naphthylamine, benzidine and 4 amino-biphenyl, are particularly associated with tumour development. β-naphthylamine is particularly important in relation to bladder cancer. Azo dyes, such as scarlet red and butter yellow are also carcinogenic and have in the past been used as dyes for foodstuffs or leather.

5. False
The preparation of tobacco and cigarettes does not hold any risk for industrial workers. The carcinogens in tobacco are coal tar products which form only when the tobacco is smoked. Nicotine is not carcinogenic.

13.7 The following infections are associated with the development of cancer:

1. Clostridial infections
2. HBV infection

3. EBV infection
4. Chlamydial infections
5. Schistosomiasis

1. False
Clostridia are Gram-positive anaerobic spore bearing organisms and are not known to have any neoplastic association. *Clostridium welchii, oedematiens* and *histolyticum* cause gas gangrene with *Cl. welchii* also causing severe food poisoning. *Clostridium tetani* causes tetanus and *Clostridium botulinus*, botulism, a severe and often fatal toxaemic disease resulting from the ingestion of contaminated food.

2. True
Hepatitis B virus is associated with the development of primary hepatoma particularly in West Africa. It also causes acute liver failure and the subacute or chronic forms of active hepatitis caused by this virus may lead to a macronodular form of cirrhosis.

3. True
The Epstein–Barr virus is a herpes virus which has been isolated from the lymphocytes of Burkitt lymphoma, a tumour of the jaw occurring principally in African children. It has also been established that individuals suffering from nasopharyngeal carcinomas in South East Asia have a high titre of antibodies to this virus.

4. False
The chlamydia are not associated with neoplastic disease. They are infectious agents about 300 nm in diameter which cause trachoma, ophthalmia neonatorum, lymphogranuloma venereum and psittacosis. They cannot be cultured on normal culture media and have to be grown in eggs or tissue culture.

5. True
The deposition of schistosome eggs in the wall of the bladder causes a metaplasia of the bladder mucosa to occur from the normal transitional cell to a squamous cell epithelium. The vesical tumours that develop in association with schistosomiasis are squamous cell carcinomas.

13.8 An increase in the frequency of malignant disease occurs in the following conditions:

1. Following the long term administration of immunosuppressive agents
2. Large bowel Crohn's disease
3. Coeliac disease
4. Ulcerative colitis
5. Xeroderma pigmentosum

1. True
Long term immunosuppressive therapy is required following renal homotransplantation. In patients in whom the graft is successfully maintained by such treatment, an increase in the incidence of all types of malignancy has now become apparent.

2. False
Malignant disease does not appear to follow long term granulomatous disease of the large bowel.

3. True
An increased incidence of malignancy has now been reported in this condition. This is believed to be caused by the loss of lymphocytes from the mucosal surface of the bowel, leading to an immunological defect in the affected individuals. An increased incidence of lymphoma has been particularly noted.

4. True
Chronic ulcerative colitis is followed by an increase in large bowel malignancy. All recorded series show that the incidence of malignancy in this disease increases with the length of the clinical history and the severity of the disease.

5. True
Xeroderma pigmentosum is a classical premalignant condition. Sufferers from this inherited disease rapidly develop skin cancer after exposure to ultra violet light.

13.9 An enhancement of tumour growth or an increased incidence of tumour formation may occur:

1. following the long term administration of immunosuppressive drugs
2. following immunological enhancement

3. due to the release of soluble antigens by the tumour cells
4. due to an alteration of T-cell function
5. due to the excessive production or release of lysosomal enzymes

1. True
An increase in the incidence of non-Hodgkin's lymphoma has been reported in patients undergoing long term immunosuppressive treatment with drugs such as azathioprine. This drug is commonly used following renal transplantation or for the treatment of autoimmune diseases such as systemic lupus erythematosus.

2. True
Immunological enhancement of tumour growth develops because of the production of 'blocking' antibody. This protects the tumour antigens from any cell-mediated immune response which the presence of the tumour provokes. In an experimental animal immunological enhancement of a transplantable tumour can be provoked by the prior immunisation of the recipient with a dead tumour extract before the injection of live tumour cells.

3. True
Tumours may shed soluble tumour specific transplantation antigens (TSTA) into the circulation which then react with the antigen reactive sites on effector T-cells thus reducing the severity of the cell-mediated immune response mounted to effect destruction of the tumour. This is one of the causes of a tumour 'sneaking through' a powerful immune response.

4. True
T-lymphocytes may exert a suppressor as well as an effector action in the body's immune response mounted against a tumour. The suppressor T-lymphocytes form a distinct sub-population differing from the effector cells and distinguished by their different surface (Ly) antigens. A balance between suppressor and effector lymphocytes forms the regulatory basis of the immune response.

5. False
Lysosomal enzymes, chiefly found in the macro-

phages, are important in degrading antigen prior to its presentation to the lymphocytes. These enzymes are mainly hydrolytic and proteolytic and thus are effective, following the activation of the macrophages by lymphokine, in destroying tumour cells and micro-organisms which have undergone phagocytosis.

13.10 The following substances are oncofoetal antigens:

1. HSA
2. α-foetoprotein
3. Bence–Jones protein
4. Chorionic gonadotrophin
5. Carcinoembryonic antigen

1. False

Human serum albumin is obviously not an oncofoetal antigen although it is frequently employed as an antigen in investigations with experimental animals.

2. True

α-fetoprotein is a globulin forming about 50 per cent of the total foetal plasma protein. It is absent after birth but is formed in over 50 per cent of patients with malignant hepatoma.

3. False

Bence–Jones proteins are free light chains of the immunoglobulin molecules that are passed in the urine in patients suffering from multiple myeloma. They may have $\varkappa$ or λ antigenic determinants. These proteins precipitate on heating the urine to 80°C but return into solution at higher temperatures.

4. False

Large amounts of chorionic gonadotrophin are produced in normal pregnancy and following the development of hydatidiform moles or choriocarcinomas. In the latter, therefore, urine pregnancy tests are strongly positive. Despite this, chorionic gonadotrophin cannot strictly be called an oncofoetal antigen.

5. True

Carcinoembryonic antigen is found in foetal cells

and in some colonic cancers. Unfortunately it is not very specific because other tumours of the gastrointestinal tract may form the antigen and it may also be formed in pregnancy and in a variety of non-neoplastic conditions including cirrhosis of the liver.

13.11 The incidence of tumours is increased in:

1. sarcoidosis
2. Wiskott–Aldrich syndrome
3. ataxia telangiectasis
4. patients treated over long periods with corticosteroids
5. patients receiving azathioprine

1. False
Despite the depression of certain parameters of T-lymphocyte function which occurs in sarcoidosis there is no evidence of any increase in the incidence of malignancy in this disease.

2. True
The Wiskott–Aldrich syndrome is a sex linked recessive disease which causes the affected children to suffer from atopic eczema, thrombocytopenia and an increased susceptibility to infection. Eventually failure of T-lymphocyte function occurs accompanied by an increased incidence of lymphomas.

3. True
Ataxia telangiectasis is an autosomal recessive condition in which the thymus is hypoplastic. Delayed hypersensitivity reactions are depressed and plasma concentrations of IgA and IgG fall. A considerable number of patients develop malignant lymphomas or lymphatic leukaemia. The disease usually presents in infancy with cerebellar ataxia due to the associated atrophy of the cerebellar cortex and demyelination of the cerebellar peduncles.

4. False
There is no evidence that prolonged treatment with corticosteroids predisposes to tumour development.

5. True
A major component of immunosuppressive therapy following renal transplantation is azathioprine. In

such patients an increased incidence of non-Hodgkin's lymphomas has now been reported.

Section 14. TUMOURS

14.1 A tumour may be defined as:

1. an abnormal mass of tissue
2. a growth of tissue which exceeds and is unco-ordinated with that of normal tissues
3. a growth of tissue which is limited and co-ordinated with that of the rest of the body
4. an abnormal increase in the cells of a tissue
5. a malformation in which the various tissues of the part are present in improper proportions or distribution

1. True
This is the opening phrase of the definition of a tumour as proposed by the late Professor R. A. Willis.

2. True
This is the second part of the definition of a tumour as constructed by Willis. It is followed by a third part, i.e. the growth of the tumour persists in the same excessive manner after cessation of the stimulus or stimuli which evoked the change.

3. False
A tissue, the growth of which is limited and co-ordinated with that of the rest of the body, is a malformation. A classic example is the cutaneous angioma, otherwise known as the 'port-wine stain' which grows only with the growth of the rest of the body and does not extend to involve a greater and greater territory of tissue.

4. False
This is the simple definition of hyperplasia. Hyperplasia usually occurs as:
(a) A compensatory response to loss of tissue of the same kind
(b) An increased functional demand which cannot be satisfied by the tissue already present
(c) Disturbed hormonal control of the activity of the tissue

5. False
This is the definition of a hamartoma.

14.2 Broder's classification of tumours attempted to classify tumours according to:

1. their origin
2. the degree of differentiation of a tumour
3. the degree of stromal response
4. the degree of lymphocytic infiltration of the tumour
5. the number of mitoses found in a given area of the tumour

1. False
Although Broder worked mainly with tumours of squamous epithelium.

2. True
This was the fundamental basis of Broder's classification. He recognised four grades of malignancy according to the degree of differentiation of the tumour. Grade 1, when more than 75 per cent of the tumour cells were differentiated; Grade 4, when less than 25 per cent of the tumour cells were differentiated with intermediate values in grades 2 and 3. This classification has been abandoned for many reasons:

(a) It is time consuming and, therefore, expensive
(b) Different parts of a tumour may show entirely different histological characteristics
(c) The results did not always correspond to the prognosis which is what Broder sought to establish. Thus a Grade 1 tumour of the skin has excellent prognosis whereas a Grade 1 bronchial carcinoma has a poor prognosis.

3. False
Stromal response, particularly of breast tumours, has been shown to influence prognosis but was not taken into account by Broder who was chiefly concerned with skin cancer.

4. False
Lymphocytic infiltration was not considered in Broder's classification although some importance is now attributed to this aspect. The degree of lymphocytic infiltration is regarded by many patholo-

gists as an indication of the body's immunological response to the tumour.

5. True
The number of mitoses indicating a greater degree of malignancy. Various modifications of Broder's original classification have been proposed one of which, applied by Greenhough to breast tumours, took into account three features of these glandular carcinomata:

(a) Tubule formation
(b) The regularity in size, shape and staining of the nuclei of the tumour cells
(c) Number of mitoses

14.3 Neoplastic disease may be associated with the following conditions:

1. Dermatomyositis
2. Acanthosis nigricans
3. Necrobiosis lipoidica
4. Thrombophlebitis migrans
5. Polyarteritis nodosa

1. True
Approximately 20 per cent of patients suffering from dermatomyositis have an underlying malignant condition. Dermatomyositis is an inflammatory lesion of muscle in which a mononuclear infiltrate occurs between the muscle bundles which themselves show mild degrees of degeneration and a loss of the normal transverse striations. The cutaneous lesions consist of erythematous patches with slight oedema. Clinically, there is muscle weakness.

2. True
Acanthosis nigricans is associated with visceral malignancy and occasionally with Hodgkin's disease or osteogenic sarcoma.

3. False
Necrobiosis lipoidica is not associated with neoplasia. It is a condition in which yellowish demarcated lesions develop on the shins, the centre of which become atrophic, breaking down to form ulcers. Histologically the lesions may be necrobiotic and

granulomatous. Diabetes is the underlying disease in approximately two thirds of affected individuals.

4. True
Thrombophlebitis migrans is chiefly associated with tumours of the pancreas, lung, stomach and female genital tract. Clinically, repeated attacks of segmental thrombosis occurs in both the superficial and the deep veins, attacks which heal spontaneously.

5. False
Polyarteritis nodosa is not associated with malignant disease but with hypersensitivity to a number of drugs including the sulphonamides and the anti-inflammatory agents such as phenylbutazone. It also occurs in HBV infections. The underlying cause is immune complex disease resulting in a necrotising arteritis affecting both deep and superficial vessels accompanied by a polymorphonuclear leucocyte infiltration around the vessels.

14.4 General phenomena associated with neoplasia may include

1. fever
2. cachexia
3. thrombotic episodes
4. polycythaemia
5. dermatomyositis

1. True
Fever, unassociated with infection, is particularly associated with the following tumours:
  (a) Nephroblastoma
  (b) Carcinoma of the renal tubules (hypernephroma)
  (c) Lymphomata
The cause of such pyrexia remains uncertain although it must be due to pyrogens formed by the breakdown products of the tumour.

2. True
Cachexia is one of the common manifestations of widespread and terminal malignancy. The cause may be difficult to identify but in gastrointestinal tumours loss of appetite, bleeding and sepsis play a part.

3. True
The classic thrombotic episode associated with neo-plasia is that described by Trousseau in 1865, of recurrent superficial and deep venous thrombosis which undergo spontaneous remission, thrombo-phlebitis migrans. Rarely, a non-bacterial thrombotic endocarditis occurs in widespread malignant disease and even rarer is disseminated intravascular coagulation.

4. True
Polycythaemia does not normally complicate neopla-sia, indeed the reverse is usually the case due either to blood loss, invasion of the red marrow or as yet unidentified causes. One exception is renal carci-noma which, by producing excessive erythropoietin, leads to a polycythaemia.

5. True
Dermatomyositis is a disorder which affects the skin, muscles and blood vessels. A coagulative necrosis occurs together with a small round cell infiltration around the smaller arteries. Approximately 30 per cent of all patients suffering from dermatomyositis between 50 and 70 years of age are found to be suffering from disseminated malignant disease usually arising from the gastrointestinal tract and less frequently the bladder and bronchus.

14.5 The following tumours may secrete hormones:

1. Carcinoid tumours
2. Choriocarcinoma
3. Arrhenoblastoma
4. Teratoma
5. Seminoma

1. False
Carcinoid tumours, if active, secrete the vasoactive material 5-hydroxytryptamine (serotonin). Such tu-mours occur in the appendix, ileum and colon aris-ing from the Kulchitsky cells. Only those tumours arising from the midgut tend to be active secre-tors. The release of 5-HT causes intermittent flushing of the face, an increase in intestinal mobility leading to diarrhoea, bronchospasm and lesions on the pul-

monary or tricuspid valves causing right sided heart failure.

2. True
Choriocarcinomas produce excessive quantities of chorionic gonadotrophin with the result that severe uterine bleeding occurs. Approximately 50 per cent follow the development of a hydatidiform mole whilst 25 per cent develop following perfectly normal pregnancies.

3. True
The arrhenoblastoma is a tumour of the ovary which commonly secretes abnormal amounts of masculinising hormones. This results in virilisation and sterility, the latter because of the cessation of ovulation.

4. True
Teratomas of the ovary may secrete either androgens or oestrogens.

5. False
Seminomas of the testes do not produce hormones.

14.6 Exfoliative cytology is useful for the diagnosis of:

1. meningioma
2. bronchial cancer
3. multiple myeloma
4. cervical cancer
5. vesical cancer

1. False
The examination of cerebro-spinal fluid for exfoliated cells has not been shown to be particularly useful in the diagnosis of tumours of the CNS. Meningiomas do not generally shed cells into the CSF.

2. True
Malignant cells can be demonstrated in the sputum, bronchial washings and if present, in a pleural effusion, in patients suffering from bronchial cancer.

3. False
Although malignant plasma cells may be demonstrated occasionally in the peripheral blood in patients with multiple myeloma, this cannot strictly be

called exfoliative cytology. Malignant cells in this condition are usually sought in marrow specimens.

4. True
Vaginal and cervical smears are commonly used to eliminate or confirm a diagnosis of carcinoma of the cervix or uterus. The abnormal cells which are pleomorphic and hyperchromatic are demonstrated by the use of a 'Papanicolaou' smear. This technique may also identify carcinoma *in-situ* and various forms of dysplasia.

5. True
Exfoliative cytology is used extensively for the exclusion or diagnosis of tumours of the bladder. It is also extensively used in the screening of asymptomatic individuals working in the aniline dye industry.

14.7 The findings of the following substances in excessive quantities in the blood may be due to the presence of a specific type of tumour:

1. Noradrenaline
2. 5-hydroxytryptamine
3. Carcinoembryonic antigen
4. Prostaglandins
5. Calcium

1. True
Excessive noradrenaline may indicate the presence of a phaeochromocytoma although this tumour also produces excessive quantities of adrenaline. The presenting symptoms of these tumours are determined by the relative concentration of the two hormones.

2. True
Excessive 5-hydroxytryptamine (serotonin) indicates the presence of a carcinoid tumour of the small bowel otherwise known as an argentaffinoma because the cytoplasm of the tumour cell can form deposits of silver from silver salts.

3. True
Carcinoembryonic antigen, one of the oncofetal antigens, is associated with gastrointestinal tumours. An estimation of this marker is of little initial assistance in their diagnosis but it is of some value as an

indicator of metastatic recurrence since above normal values suggests that hepatic metastases have developed.

4. False
Although prostaglandins are found in a variety of tissues such as the seminal vesicles, lung, iris and renal medulla no tumour has been described in which this group of compounds is produced in excessive quantities.

5. True
Hypercalcaemia may indicate the presence of a benign or malignant parathyroid tumour or more commonly the presence of extensive osseous metastases. The latter arise most commonly from primary tumours of the breast, thyroid, bronchus, kidney or prostate.

14.8 Neuroblastomas are most common in:

1. children
2. adults
3. the adrenal medulla
4. the floor of the fourth ventricle
5. sympathetic ganglia

1. True
These tumours now classified as sympatheticoblastoma only occur in infancy. Two overlapping syndromes have been described. Pepper's associated with hepatomegaly and Hutchinson's associated with osseous metastases in the orbit which lead to periorbital bruising and exophthalmos.

2. False
Although occasionally neuroblastoma may mature into nerve fibres and cells forming ganglioneuromata.

3. True
The commonest site of origin of this tumour is the adrenal medulla. Histological examination reveals that the tumour is composed of tightly packed masses of darkly-staining round cells which are sometimes arranged in rosette-like clusters.

4. False
Tumours arising from the floor of the fourth ventricle

near the cerebellum are another developmental tumour, the medulloblastoma.

5. True
Neuroblastoma may arise from the sympathetic ganglia but this site is not as common as the adrenal medulla.

14.9 Hormone dependency may be exhibited by the following tumours:

1. Malignant melanoma
2. Prostatic carcinoma
3. Follicular carcinoma of the thyroid
4. Bronchial carcinoma
5. Retinoblastoma

1. True
Although hormone therapy has no beneficial effect on malignant melanoma well documented reports do appear in the literature of such tumours regressing during pregnancy, presumably due to its hormonal effects.

2. True
The scientific basis of hormone dependency was first established by Charles Huggins of Chicago after the Second World War when he discovered that carcinoma of the prostate was affected by altering its hormonal environment. Later he discovered that oophorectomy and adrenalectomy had a beneficial effect on disseminated breast cancer. It is interesting to note, however, that Beatson and others in the early part of this century had observed that the former operation sometimes produced great, although temporary, improvement in advanced breast cancer.

3. True
The growth of both follicular and papillary tumours of the thyroid may be suppressed by the administration of thyroxine.

4. False
Bronchial carcinomata are not hormone dependent although they occasionally produce hormones, in

particular ACTH. When this occurs Cushingoid features develop.

5. False
This is a tumour of infancy of which about six per cent of cases are familial. There is no evidence of hormone dependency.

14.10 The commonest tumours of the central nervous system arise from:

1. the meninges
2. primary tumours elsewhere in the body
3. neuroglia
4. the blood vessels
5. nerve cells

1. False
Meningioma, developing from the arachnoid cells which lie in the deep surface of the dura, are only the third commonest tumour of the central nervous system.

2. True
Secondary metastatic deposits are the commonest tumours of the central nervous system. The tumours which most commonly metastasise to the central nervous system arise from the breast, bronchus and the melanocytes.

3. True
Tumours of the neuroglia are known as gliomas. These are the commonest primary tumours of the central nervous system. This group includes the astrocytomas, ependymomas and oligodendrogliomas.

4. False
True tumours of the blood vessels of the brain are rare. Hamartomatous malformations form about 2 per cent of cerebral tumours.

5. False
In childhood, usually below the age of four, medulloblastomas are found in the region of the fourth ventricle near the cerebellum. In adults primary nerve cell tumours such as ganglioneuroma and ganglioglioma are rare.

243

14.11 The 'doubling time' of a malignant tumour is affected by a number of factors including:

1. tumour necrosis
2. exfoliation
3. the percentage of cells in the resting phase
4. the oxygen content of the tumour cells environment
5. nuclear size

1. True
The degree of necrosis affects the total number of malignant cells in a tumour which are capable of division. Necrosis is precipitated by an inadequate blood supply and in relation to epithelial tumours of the gastrointestinal tract, infection.

2. True
Exfoliation is also a significant factor leading to a loss of tumour cells capable of division. This feature is particularly important in tumours of the gastrointestinal tract and the urothelium.

3. True
The proportion of cells in the resting phase varies considerably in different cell systems. The percentage of resting cells may vary between 20 and 50 per cent of the whole in normal bone marrow.

In malignant tumours the condition is more complicated because of their heterogeneous nature. Thus some clones of cells in a tumour are capable of only four or five divisions before dying.

4. True
Although the cell cycle time remains the same in hypoxic conditions the dividing fraction of cells increases as the oxygen content of the environment rises.

5. False
Nuclear size bears no relationship to the time taken for the division of malignant cells.

14.12 The interphase is:

1. situated between the prophase and metaphase
2. a resting stage between cell division
3. associated with growth of a cell

4. accompanied by the accumulation of RNA
5. situated between the anaphase and the telophase

1. False
The prophase may be regarded as the beginning of cell division. During this phase the chromosomes become visible and during the metaphase the spindle is formed radiating from the centrioles situated at opposite poles of the cell.

2. True
During the interphase chromosomes cannot be detected within the nucleus as discrete structures by a light microscope.

3. True
The interphase is associated with the accumulation of ribonucleic acid in the cell.

4. True

5. False
The interphase follows the telophase during which the chromosomes elongate and disappear as the new nuclear membrane forms and the spindle disappears.

14.13 The embryonic tumours of infancy include:

1. nephroblastoma
2. osteogenic sarcoma (osteosarcoma)
3. medulloblastoma
4. cholangiocarcinoma
5. lympho-epithelioma

1. True
This renal neoplasm may appear as a rapidly growing tumour, 80 per cent occurring under age four. Known also as a Wilm's tumour it accounts for approximately eight per cent of childhood malignancies. This tumour spreads rapidly by the blood stream producing metastases in the lungs. Microscopically it is composed of a mass of spindle-shaped cells in which acini and tubules are found.

2. False
Osteogenic sarcoma (osteosarcoma) arises from the cells of the primitive bone-forming mesenchyme. It is the commonest primary malignant tumour of bone

excluding myeloma. Seventy-five per cent of sufferers are between 10 and 25 years of age but a similar tumour also occurs in older patients suffering from Paget's disease of bone.

3. True
These tumours develop in the cerebellum forming a soft greyish-white mass which commonly protrudes into the fourth ventricle and spreads over the surface of the brain in a thin sheet to obscure the normal convoluted surface. Microscopically they are composed of spherical or cylindrical cells which have little cytoplasm and no fibrils. Rosettes occur without a central cavity.

4. False
These rare tumours develop from the cells of the biliary epithelium and are less common than true hepatocellular carcinoma. These tumours are commonest in the Far East, in which the majority are associated with infestation of the liver flukes.

5. False
An anaplastic squamous carcinoma heavily infiltrated with lymphocytes. This tumour is particularly common in adult Chinese in whom it is commonly associated with a high titre of antibody to the Epstein–Barr virus.

14.14 The following tumours may produce hormones:

1. Choriocarcinoma
2. Bronchial carcinoma
3. Fibroma of the ovary
4. Islet cell tumours of the pancreas
5. Chromophobe pituitary adenoma

1. True
Choriocarcinoma frequently produces chorionic gonadotrophins in much greater concentrations than are found in a normal pregnancy. This is an important prognostic feature since failure of the hormonal level to fall to normal following excision or treatment of the primary tumour by chemotherapy indicates tumour tissue is still present.

2. True

A bronchial carcinoma may be associated with ectopic hormone production. The commonest hormone produced is ACTH leading to the development of Cushingoid features.

3. False

Benign fibroma of the ovary does not produce any hormonal disturbance but large tumours of this type may be associated with wasting, ascites and right sided hydrothorax, Meig's syndrome.

4. True

According to the cell of origin islet cell tumours of the pancreas can secrete excessive quantities of insulin leading to intermittent hypoglycaemia or excessive gastrin leading to the Zollinger–Ellison syndrome.

5. True

Normally chromophobe adenomata produce their pathological effects by pressure and only occasionally is a hormone secreted by the tumour itself. Destruction of the anterior hypophysis by such a tumour, however, produces progressive panhypopituitarism, pressure on the optic chiasma, a bitemporal hemianopia and by destruction of the hypothalamus, diabetes insipidus. If hormone production does occur, growth hormone, prolactin or ACTH may be produced.

Section 15: VIRAL DISEASES

15.1 The following are viral diseases:

1. Cytomegalic inclusion disease
2. Trachoma
3. Dengue
4. Primary atypical pneumonia
5. Typhus

1. True

Cytomegalic inclusion disease is caused by the cytomegalovirus which is a ubiquitous herpes virus. It causes disease chiefly in immunodeficient states and affects mainly the lungs and bronchial mucosa although a feature is the development of widespread large intranuclear inclusion bodies. These can be found in the salivary glands, pancreas, liver and kidneys.

2. False

Trachoma is caused by a subgroup of the chlamydia, a group of obligate intracellular organisms 300 nm in diameter. One group of serotypes is responsible for hyperendemic trachoma which is a major cause of blindness in Africa and Asia. Another group cause urethritis and cervicitis. This is particularly important because ophthalmia neonatorum is acquired during the passage of the infants through the infected birth canal.

3. True

Dengue is an acute painful febrile illness which is often haemorrhagic. It is produced by an RNA virus of the togavirus type. The virus is arthropod borne (Arbor) and transmitted by the mosquito *Aedes aegypti*. The dengue virus is related to that causing yellow fever.

4. False

Primary atypical pneumonia is caused by the *Mycoplasma pneumoniae* which are 200 to 250 nm in diameter and among the smallest of bacteria. Patients with mycoplasmal pneumonia have autoantibodies against the I antigen carried on erythrocytes.

5. False

Epidemic typhus which is transmitted by the louse, is caused by the *Rickettsia prowazeki*, obligate intracellular parasites that can be grown in tissue culture or eggs. The rickettsiae are small organisms 300 to 700 nm diameter. Other rickettsiae cause similar febrile illnesses and are either flea or tick borne.

15.2 Encephalitis may be a complication of the following virus infections:

1. Epstein–Barr virus
2. Measles virus
3. Rubella virus
4. Herpes virus
5. Adenovirus

1. True

EBV is the cause of infectious mononucleosis (glandular fever).

2. True

Measles is only occasionally associated with a transient encephalitis. More especially it is the cause of subacute sclerosing panencephalitis (SSPE). This condition is thought to arise because of a failure of specific cell-mediated immunity towards the virus and is associated with high antibody levels.

3. True

A progressive encephalitis may occur in children with the congenital rubella syndrome.

4. True

Herpes simplex infection may be associated with meningo-encephalitis, particularly in immunodepressed individuals.

5. False

The adenoviruses chiefly affect the upper respiratory tract and occasionally cause gastroenteritis. They are not particularly associated with the development of encephalitis.

15.3 Inclusion bodies are found in the following viral infections:

1. Zoster
2. Yellow fever
3. Rabies
4. Hepatitis B
5. Smallpox

1. True

In zoster, as in herpes simplex, giant cells containing intranuclear inclusion bodies can be found in the epidermis. These occupy most of the nucleus except for a peripheral clear zone separating them from the nuclear membrane.

2. False

Yellow fever is an arbovirus infection not associated with obvious inclusion bodies.

3. True

Rabies is caused by rhabdoviruses. The pathognomonic histological feature of this disease is the development of acidophilic cytoplasmic inclusion bodies known as Negri bodies in the neurones, particularly in the pyramidal cells of the hippocampus and in the Purkinje cells in the cerebellum.

4. False

Intracellular inclusion bodies are not found in infections due to the hepatitis B virus. However, actual HBV particles may be found in the serum by electron microscopy.

5. True

Both smallpox and vaccinia are associated with the development of spheroidal eosinophilic masses in the cytoplasm of the epidermal cells known as the Guanieri bodies. Within them the elementary particles of the virus which contain DNA are elaborated.

15.4 The following are RNA containing viruses:

1. Rhinovirus
2. Herpes virus
3. Vaccinia
4. Yellow fever
5. Influenza

1. True

Rhinoviruses are upper respiratory tract viruses causing the common cold. They are a subgroup of the picornaviruses, a group which also include the enteroviruses. Their habitat is the nose and they are amongst the smallest of all viruses infecting man.

2. False

The herpes viruses cause herpes simplex, varicella/zoster, cytomegalic inclusion disease and infectious mononucleosis. They are DNA viruses with a capsid of cubical symmetry possessing no outer envelope. Among the most interesting members of this group is the Epstein–Barr virus which is the cause of infectious mononucleosis and is also found in children suffering from Burkitt's lymphoma in Central Africa.

3. False

Vaccinia is a large brick shaped DNA containing virus belonging to the group known as the poxviruses. Included in this group is also the virus responsible for small pox.

4. True
Yellow fever is caused by an RNA containing togavirus, most of which are arthropod borne, hence the collective name for the group, the ARBOR viruses.

5. True
The Influenza virus is an RNA myxovirus. The capsid has a helical symmetry and an outer envelope. This group of viruses undergo frequent antigenic variations making it difficult to prepare effective vaccines. Epidemic influenza is caused by the subgroup Influenza A.

15.5 The Epstein–Barr virus is associated with:

1. glandular fever
2. the Australia antigen
3. Burkitt's lymphoma
4. nasopharyngeal carcinoma
5. the common cold

1. True
The Epstein–Barr virus (EBV) is a herpes virus. It is definitely associated with glandular fever since the peripheral lymphocytes in patients suffering from this disease can be shown to contain the virus. Furthermore, during the acute phase of the illness antibodies to EBV can be identified in the patient's serum. In addition individuals suffering from infectious mononucleosis also develop heterophile antibodies in the serum which are capable of agglutinating sheep erythrocytes; such antibodies are not absorbed by guinea-pig kidney but can be absorbed with ox erythrocytes, the basis of the Paul Bunnell test.

2. False
The Australia antigen is not associated with infection by the EBV. It is associated, however, with the hepatitis B virus and is the name originally given to HBsAg because this antigen was originally identified in the serum of an Australian aborigine.

3. True
The EBV was first isolated from cultures of lympho-

blasts in children suffering from Burkitt's lymphoma, a tumour affecting the jaws and facial region of children in Central Africa. It is especially prevalent in malaria endemic areas possibly because chronic malarial infection reduces immunity to the virus. An unexplained finding is the relatively low titre of anti-EBV antibodies found in Burkitt's lymphoma.

4. True
Nasopharyngeal carcinoma is associated with a high titre of antibodies to EBV.

5. False
The common cold is associated with rhinoviruses, a subgroup of the picornaviruses.

15.6 The hepatitis B virus:

1. is transmitted by the oral route
2. is transmitted by dogs
3. is common in renal dialysis units
4. is the cause of Burkitt's lymphoma
5. causes immune complex disease

1. True
Hepatitis B virus (HBV) is a DNA virus transmitted by the oral–faecal route, by aerosols or by syringe and needle. An HBV infection can be detected by identifying the antigen HBsAg in the serum of carriers.

2. False
There does not appear to be an intermediate host. However, in the tropics a mosquito vector has been suspected.

3. True
Renal dialysis units are high risk areas for HBV infection as infection is common in people with chronic renal failure. A number of renal units have been associated with a high mortality among doctors and nursing staff from HBV infection. Other groups in which HBV is common are in mental hospitals and drug addicts.

4. False
Burkitt's lymphoma is associated with EB virus in-

fection. HBV infection has, however, been associated with primary hepatoma particularly in the tropics.

5. True
HBV infection may be associated with polyarteritis nodosa and arthritis. Immunoglobulin and complement have both been demonstrated in the walls of blood vessels and immune complexes containing HBV have been demonstrated as aggregates in the serum of infected individuals by electron microscopy.

15.7 The following infections may be successfully prevented by the administration of a vaccine:

1. Herpes simplex
2. Rabies
3. Lassa fever
4. Poliomyelitis
5. Yellow fever

1. False
No effective vaccine exists against infection by the herpes viruses. Herpes simplex is an infection in which the virus may remain latent for much of the time, probably in nerve cells.

2. True
An effective vaccine against rabies was first produced by Pasteur in the form of an attenuated virus. The risk associated with this and other similar nervous tissue vaccines is of inducing an autoimmune allergic encephalomyelitis. Modern anti-rabies vaccine is prepared from duck embryos and does not carry such a high rate of neurological complications. Recently a vaccine grown in human diploid fibroblasts has been introduced which appears to cause even fewer neurological complications.

3. False
There is no effective vaccine against Lassa fever which is caused by a virus of the arenavirus group which is prevalent in West Africa.

4. True
The original Salk vaccine was a formolised dead

vaccine administered by injection. The currently used Sabin vaccine is an attenuated vaccine given by the oral route.

5. True
An effective vaccine which maintains its effect for six years can be produced by using the 17D strain which is attenuated by mouse passage and grown in chick embryos.

15.8 The following viral infections are controlled by cell-mediated immunity:

1. Herpes simplex
2. Cytomegalic inclusion disease
3. Poliomyelitis
4. ECHO virus
5. Vaccinia

1. True
The herpes simplex virus can cause severe generalised visceral disease in children born with a primary T-lymphocyte deficiency.

2. True
This ubiquitous virus causes a disseminated infection which particularly affects the upper respiratory tract of babies with T-lymphocyte deficiency, adults receiving immunosuppressive drugs and individuals in whom cell-mediated immunity has diminished due to the development of Hodgkin's disease.

3. False
The polioviruses are classified as picornaviruses, subgroup A; among which are the enteroviruses and the rhinoviruses, the polioviruses belonging to the former. It is believed that natural protection is produced by an IgA antibody which is secreted by the gut associated lymphoid tissue. For this reason immunisation is most effective when carried out by the oral administration of the appropriate vaccine.

4. False
The ECHO viruses are a subgroup of the picornaviruses, the name standing for 'enteric cytopathogenic human orphan'. This group is responsible for a

variety of febrile illnesses including meningitis, respiratory infections, conjunctivitis and diarrhoea. As with the polioviruses it is believed that natural protection is dependent upon the production of an IgA antibody by the gastrointestinal tract.

5. True
The 'reaction of immunity' to vaccinia virus is a delayed hypersensitivity reaction seen when the individual is vaccinated on the second or subsequent occasions. This reaction is T-lymphocyte mediated as is resistance to clinical infection. The presence of immunity is marked by the failure of the individual to develop a 'pock' at the vaccination site.

15.9 Interferon:

1. is a complement component
2. may be induced by bacterial endotoxin
3. may be induced by Poly I:C
4. is a dialysable factor
5. is species-specific

1. False
Interferon is not a serum protein. It is secreted by a number of cells throughout the body, particularly lymphocytes and is frequently classified as a lymphokine.

2. True
Interferon can be produced in a number of tissue culture systems, one of which is lymphocytes incubated with bacterial endotoxin or plant mitogens, such as phytohaemagglutinin.

3. True
Poly I:C, a complex of polyinosinic acid and polycytidilic acid, is a synthetic double stranded RNA molecule which acts as an artificial inducer of interferon production.

4. False
Interferon is a protein variously estimated as between 20 000 and 160 000 molecular weight. It will not, therefore, pass through a dialysis membrane.

5. True
Interferon is species-specific. Thus a chick cell prepa-

ration is active in chick cells but much less effective in mouse cells. Similarly interferon active in human infections must be produced in cultures of human or primate cells. Thus although a potentially important therapeutic agent its production presents practical obstacles.

15.10 The following diseases are caused by chlamydia:

1. Yellow fever
2. Lymphogranuloma venereum
3. Mumps
4. Psittacosis
5. Herpes simplex

1. False
Yellow fever is caused by an arthropod borne RNA virus of the togavirus group. It is transmitted by the mosquito, *Aedes aegypti*.

2. True
Lymphogranuloma venereum is caused by a subgroup A chlamydia which is closely related to the chlamydia causing trachoma. The Frei test for LGV is a delayed hypersensitivity skin test.

3. False
Mumps is caused by a paramyxovirus. Typically a bilateral parotitis occurs but in addition there is a high incidence of involvement of central nervous system and occasionally orchitis. Paramyxoviruses are large filamentous double stranded, RNA viruses (150 to 220 nm in size).

4. True
Psittacosis is a febrile disease chiefly involving the respiratory tract, caused by a subgroup B chlamydia. It is acquired by inhaling infected aerosols or dust from birds, usually of domestic origin.

5. False
Herpes viruses are double stranded DNA viruses which produce acidophilic intranuclear inclusion bodies. The herpes viruses have the peculiar property of remaining latent for many months or years and then being reactivated by a variety of stimuli,

including UV light and febrile illnesses. The herpes group also includes varicella/zoster, the Epstein–Barr virus and cytomegalovirus.

Section 16. VASCULAR CONDITIONS

16.1 The chief pathological changes of atherosclerosis are:

1. deposition of lipid in the smooth muscle cells of the intima
2. fragmentation of the internal elastic lamina
3. calcification
4. contraction of the vessel
5. collagen deposition

1. True
It is the initial deposition of lipid in the smooth muscle cells, macrophages and 'foam' cells which produces the earliest detectable macroscopic changes in the arteries of the intima known as the 'fatty streak'.

2. True
Fragmentation of the internal elastic lamina causes gradually increasing weakness of the arterial wall which is followed by dilatation and aneurysm formation.

3. True
Calcification occurs in the fibrous plaques which develop within the intimal layer. These plaques contain large quantities of cholesteryl ester resembling that of the plasma lipoprotein. Calcification is not so pronounced, however, as in the condition known as Monckeberg's sclerosis.

4. False
Decrease in the lumen of an atherosclerotic artery does not occur, because of contraction of the vessel, but follows encroachment by the increasing size of the fibrous plaques or intimal rupture followed by thrombosis.

5. True
During the stage at which fibrous plaques are forming in the wall of the artery large amounts of collagen

are deposited in the wall of the artery. In the wall of a normal artery the ratio of collagen to protein is 1:4 whereas in the calcified plaques this ratio may be reduced by an increase in the absolute amount of collagen to less than 1:2.

16.2 Cholesterol is believed to be of great importance in the development of atherosclerosis because:

1. low plasma cholesterol concentrations are associated with relative freedom from atherosclerotic heart disease
2. high concentrations of cholesterol occur in the atherosclerotic plaques
3. patients suffering from steatorrhoea develop atherosclerosis at a younger age than normal individuals
4. diabetes is associated with an increased incidence of atherosclerosis
5. atherosclerosis can be induced in non-human primates by dietary measures which increase the concentration of cholesterol in the plasma

1. True
This has been well established in numerous epidemiological studies.

2. True
Between one third and one half of the calcium-free dry weight of an atherosclerotic plaque is composed of lipid of which more than 70 per cent is cholesterol.

3. False
Patients suffering from steatorrhoea have either normal or subnormal plasma concentrations of cholesterol and theoretically the development of atherosclerosis should be delayed.

4. False
Although diabetes is associated with an increased incidence of atherosclerosis this is not due to the attendant hypercholesterolaemia but probably to the hypertriglyceridaemia.

5. True
Atherosclerosis can be induced by high cholesterol containing diets in both rabbits and non-human primates.

16.3 The following conditions are associated with hyperlipidaemia:

1. Familial hypercholesterolaemia
2. The nephrotic syndrome
3. Cushing's syndrome
4. Hyperaldosteronism
5. Thyrotoxicosis

1. True
Familial hypercholesterolaemia is an autosomal dominant disease associated with an increase in type IIA and type IIB hyperlipidaemia.

2. True
Nephrosis is accompanied by an increase in type V and type IV lipids. The former consists of an excess of chylomicrons as well as pre-β-lipoproteins.

3. True
Cushing's syndrome is associated with pre-β and β-lipoprotein excess.

4. False
This hormonal disturbance has no effect on the plasma lipoprotein concentration.

5. False
Thyrotoxicosis is not associated with lipoprotein disturbance unlike hypothyroidism.

16.4 Gangrene is necrosis together with:

1. desiccation
2. colliquative necrosis
3. involvement of a limb
4. infection of the tissues with Gram-positive organisms
5. putrefaction

1. False
Although the clinician refers to dry gangrene when infarction followed by desiccation has occurred, the pathologist does not recognise this as gangrene. The change in colour in 'dry gangrene' is due to alterations in the haemoglobin of the red cells trapped in the infarcted tissues.

2. False

Colliquative necrosis may well occur in gangrene but this is not essential to the pathological definition.

3. False

Gangrene occurs in many places other than a limb, e.g. around the mouth, in the abdominal wall and in the perineum.

4. False

The bacteria responsible for the specific condition of gas gangrene are Gram-positive but the commoner surgical forms of gangrene are caused by Gram-negative organisms.

5. True

Necrosis with superadded putrefaction is the accepted pathological definition of gangrene. The responsible organisms are saprophytic, i.e. grow on decaying organic matter. The organisms concerned include the clostridia (Gram-positive), the bacterioides (Gram-negative) and fusobacterium (Gram-negative).

16.5 Infarction may occur as a complication in the following diseases:

1. Atherosclerosis
2. Monckeberg's sclerosis
3. Benign hypertension
4. Sickle-cell anaemia
5. Idiopathic thrombocytopenic purpura

1. True

Infarction may occur in any organ or tissue supplied by an atherosclerotic artery. It is caused by the sudden obstruction to the blood flow by occlusion of the lumen of the artery. This follows a subintimal haemorrhage in the wall of the diseased artery or thrombosis upon the intimal plaque. Typical infarcts of this nature occur in the heart, brain and limbs.

2. False

This is a condition affecting the major arteries of the lower limb in elderly people caused by dystrophic calcification of the media. The intima is unaffected and the lumen of the artery remains of normal diameter unless coincidental atherosclerotic changes have also occurred in the involved blood vessels.

3. False
Hypertension does not lead to infarction unless accompanied by atherosclerosis. In the brain hypertension may be associated with the development of microaneurysms of the deep penetrating arteries. These tend to rupture causing cerebral haemorrhage.

4. True
Sickle cell anaemia is frequently complicated by vascular occlusive episodes which lead to infarcts in the lungs, spleen, bone, liver or intestine. In severe cases these episodes occur within the first few years of life but they do not occur in the newborn, however severe the disease, because of the high complement of fetal haemoglobin and low percentage of HbS in the erythrocytes.

5. False
ITP occurs chiefly in children and young adults and is frequently a self-limiting disease which improves within three months. This condition is associated with bleeding from the endometrium, kidneys or gastrointestinal tract if the platelet count is below 20 000 per μml.

16.6 Liquefaction associated with necrosis occurs after infarction of the:

1. heart
2. kidney
3. brain
4. liver
5. spleen

1. False
2. False
3. True
4. False
5. False

In the heart, kidney, liver and spleen coagulative necrosis occurs. The necrotic area becomes swollen, firm, dull and lustreless. Histologically the outlines of the dead cells are usually visible under a light microscope and the dead tissue becomes firm because of the action of tissue thromboplastins on fibrinogen which, together with other plasma proteins, diffuse from the damaged membranes of the necrotic cells.

In contrast brain tissue, which has a large fluid component, becomes 'softened' when necrotic and finally turns into a turbid liquid. The histolgical architecture of the affected tissue is lost. This is colliquative necrosis.

16.7 The investigations performed in a patient suffering from Raynaud's phenomenon should include:

1. assay of haemagglutinating antibodies
2. rheumatoid factor
3. antimitochondrial antibodies
4. serum potassium
5. X-ray of the root of the neck

1. True
This investigation may reveal the presence of cold agglutinins which by agglutinating the red cells in the digital circulation cause Raynaud's phenomenon.

2. True
Rheumatoid arthritis may be associated with or mimic Raynaud's phenomenon. The serum in the majority of patients suffering from rheumatoid disease contains an IgM immunoglobulin which is an auto-antibody reacting with the patient's own IgG. This factor is normally detected by the use of the Waaler–Rose test.

3. False
Antimitochondrial antibodies are found in a number of autoimmune conditions including Hashimoto's disease of the thyroid, known also as lymphadenoid goitre or autoimmune thyroiditis. They are not found associated with Raynaud's phenomenon.

4. False
The serum potassium remains normal in all conditions associated with the Raynaud's phenomenon.

5. True
Raynaud's phenomenon may be associated with a cervical rib. If present, such a rib injures the subcla-

vian artery and causes intimal thrombosis. Embolisation from this thrombus may then cause the vascular changes associated with Raynaud's phenomenon.

16.8 Acquired syphilis of the cardiovascular system may involve the following lesions:

1. Myocardial gummata
2. Aortitis
3. Aortic regurgitation
4. Abdominal aortic aneurysm
5. Stenosis of the coronary ostia

1. True
Gummata are ubiquitous, occurring in any tissue of the body. A second type of myocardial lesion has been described in which only fibrosis occurs. There is, however, doubt as to whether this represents a specific form of syphilitic involvement.

2. True
The distinctive features of syphilitic aortitis, which is often accompanied by atherosclerosis, are as follows:
  (a) Bluish grey or porcelain-grey intimal plaques
  (b) Wrinkling and puckering of the inner aspect of the aorta with a tendency to form radial or parallel grooves, the latter in the long axis of the aorta
  (c) Sharp transverse demarcation of the aortic lesions ending at the origins of the vessels of the neck, at the level of the diaphragm or at the origin of the renal arteries
  (d) Localisation of the most extensive lesions to the ascending aorta above the sinuses of Valsalva

3. True
Aortic regurgitation occurs, not because of direct valvular involvement but because of the extension of the luetic aortitis to the valve commissures and cusps.

4. False
Syphilitic aneurysms commonly involve the arch of the aorta.

5. True
Stenosis of the coronary ostia is frequently associated

with aortic insufficiency. Stenosis occurs because of the proximal extension of the syphilitic aortic involvement.

16.9 Coarctation of the aorta is associated with:

1. a primary developmental anomaly of the third left aortic arch
2. the development of a collateral circulation to overcome the effects of the stenosis
3. strong femoral pulses
4. hypertension
5. erosion of the upper borders of the ribs

1. False
The embryological abnormality involves the fourth left aortic arch.

2. True
Massive collaterals develop, sometimes limited to within the chest, but in other cases palpable from the surface.

3. False
The femoral pulses may well be impalpable; in contrast the suprasternal and supraclavicular pulses are strong.

4. False
The hypertension found in coarctation is limited to the upper extremities, the blood pressure in the lower limbs being normal or depressed.

5. False
The erosions involve the lower borders of the ribs, usually from the third to the tenth, usually on both sides and in their posterior portions.

16.10 The following congenital anomalies of the heart are accompanied by continuous cyanosis:

1. Complete transposition of the great vessels
2. Uncomplicated patent ductus arteriosus
3. Coarctation of the aorta
4. Double aortic arch
5. Tetralogy of Fallot

1. True
This is one of the leading causes of death from cyanotic heart disease of congenital origin. The aorta arises entirely from the right ventricle and the pulmonary artery from the left.

2. False
In children suffering from uncomplicated patent ductus arteriosus blood at the high pressure in the aorta is shunted into the pulmonary artery during both systole and diastole. The pulmonary blood flow is above normal and the pulmonary artery becomes dilated, cyanosis does not develop until heart failure occurs although occasionally a reversal of flow with venous-arterial shunting may occur during crying or coughing.

3. False
Cyanosis does not occur in this condition. A striking collateral circulation develops but if this is inadequate congestive heart failure develops due to the severe obstruction to blood flow.

4. False
Symptoms from a double aortic arch are often absent. If they occur they consist of dysphagia and dyspnoea.

5. True
This combination of cardiac abnormalities is always associated with cyanosis and accounts for the majority of infants suffering from cyanotic heart disease.

16.11 Acute heart failure occurs:

1. in rheumatic fever
2. in rheumatoid arthritis
3. in myxoedema
4. following myocardial infarction
5. in acute nephritis

1. True
In acute rheumatic fever the pericardium, myocardium and the valves may be affected. In the presence of pericarditis or valvular disease one can virtually assume that myocardial involvement has occurred and evidence of right and left heart failure are commonly observed in children. Cardiac enlarge-

265

ment may occur rapidly in active rheumatic disease. The characteristic lesion is the Aschoff body which when fully developed shows hyaline change in the collagen bundles surrounded by an infiltrate of lymphocytes, macrophages and occasional polymorphonuclear cells. These occur more commonly on the left side of the heart and are especially abundant beneath the endocardium of the left atrium just above the mitral cusp. In addition to this specific lesion diffuse polymorphonuclear and lymphocytic infiltration occurs along the connective tissue planes associated with inflammatory oedema.

2. False
Rheumatoid arthritis has no effect on the heart.

3. False
Although the heart shadow is seen to be enlarged in myxoedema on plain radiographs this is chiefly due to the development of a pericardial effusion. Heart failure does not occur unless there is associated intrinsic heart disease.

4. True
Acute heart failure occurs following severe myocardial infarction due to the reduction in cardiac output resulting from the myocardial injury or because of the development of ventricular fibrillation.

5. True
Acute nephritis may be followed by heart failure due to the development of severe hypertension associated with this disease. This causes left ventricular failure.

16.12 Left sided heart failure occurs as a complication of:

1. hypertension
2. mitral regurgitation
3. pulmonary fibrosis
4. uncomplicated coronary atherosclerosis
5. tricuspid stenosis

1. True
Hypertension, depending upon its severity and the rapidity of its onset, places an increasing strain on

the myocardium and inevitably left sided heart failure develops.

2. True
Mitral regurgitation, when it is severe enough to become symptomatic, is associated with palpitations and dyspnoea. In severe cases dyspnoea on slight exertion occurs accompanied by increasing fatigue. In some patients no important manifestations of the condition occur but even so in some of these patients rapidly progressive cardiac failure may develop particularly if a bacterial endocarditis occurs.

3. False
Pulmonary fibrosis places a strain on the right side of the heart.

4. True
Uncomplicated coronary atherosclerosis is asymptomatic. Symptoms will only develop when the disease is sufficiently severe to lead to myocardial fibrosis.

5. False
Tricuspid stenosis is associated with right-sided heart failure.

16.13 A myocardial infarct may be associated with:

1. hypotension
2. a fall in the plasma GOT
3. endocardial thrombosis
4. a red infarct
5. atrial rather than ventricular fibrillation

1. True
A severe myocardial infarct causes a dramatic fall in cardiac output and so 'cardiogenic shock'.

2. False
Since the enzyme glutamic oxaloacetic transaminase is present in heart muscle myocardial necrosis leads to the liberation of this enzyme and an increase in its concentration in the blood. GOT estimations are, therefore, diagnostically useful. Elevated levels which reach a peak within 2 to 3 days are found within 6 to 12 hours of infarction.

3. True

When the infarct involves the endocardium some thrombosis is almost inevitable. This leads to the possibility of an embolic complication although this is not very common.

4. False

Because the myocardium has only a single arterial supply via the coronary vessels, a pale infarct occurs. No visible changes occur in the dead muscle for 8 hours or more. Therefore, in patients dying within a few hours neither with the naked eye nor under the light microscope can changes be seen.

5. False

The arrhythmia commonly associated with myocardial infarction is ventricular fibrillation. Because the fibrillating ventricle cannot expel blood from its cavity in sufficient volume to sustain life sudden death may follow even a minor infarct.

Section 17. HAEMATOLOGY

17.1 A low mean corpuscular haemoglobin concentration occurs in the following:

1. Iron deficiency anaemia
2. Pernicious anaemia
3. The anaemia associated with infestation with the fish tapeworm *Diphyllobothrium latum*
4. The anaemia following extensive gastric resection
5. Sideroblastic anaemia

1. True

Iron deficiency arising from a decreased intake of iron or chronic blood loss leads to a reduction in the MCHC. The common causes of chronic blood loss in the Western World include severe haemorrhoids or menorrhagia. In tropical countries ankylostomiasis is one of the commonest causes of alimentary blood loss.

2. False

The MCHC is normal. The macrocytic red cells vary in shape and size and are well filled with haemoglobin in the absence of a co-existent iron deficiency.

3. False
Diphyllobothrium latum, the fish tapeworm, is common in Scandinavian countries. Infestation causes a pure vitamin B_{12} deficiency by the deviation of the vitamin from the host to the parasite.

4. True
Extensive gastric resection may be followed by an anaemia in which the MCHC falls because both vitamin B_{12} and iron absorption may be disturbed.

5. False
This type of anaemia may be congenital (rare) or acquired. The MCHC is not markedly depressed and the plasma iron is raised, the latter helping to distinguish this condition from iron deficiency anaemia. Several drugs have been implicated as causes of acquired sideroblastic anaemia, including isoniazid, paraminosalicyclic acid, paracetamol and phenacetin.

17.2 Alterations in the structure of the Hb molecule give rise to the following diseases:

1. Haemolytic disease of the newborn
2. Sickle cell anaemia
3. Paroxysmal cold haemoglobinuria
4. Paroxysmal nocturnal haemoglobinuria
5. Thalassaemia major

1. False
This condition is due to the stimulation of maternal antibody production by an antigen possessed by the fetus and is unrelated to the actual structure of the haemoglobin molecule. The common situation is of a mother Rh-d carrying a fetus Rh-D. Isoimmunisation initially occurs in the immediate post-partum phase of placental separation in the first pregnancy. The mother is then sensitised. Any subsequent pregnancy in which the fetus is Rh positive leads to recurrent antibody production. Haemolysis of the fetal red cells is then brought about by the transplacental passage of maternal antibody into the fetal circulation.

2. True
Sickle-cell anaemia is a hereditary condition of Negroes transmitted by an autosome. The homozyg-

ous condition gives rise to the severe sickle-cell disease, the heterozygous condition the sickle-cell trait. The abnormal haemoglobin is known as Hb-S which reduced in a low oxygen tension becomes insoluble. This causes the red cells to assume a bizarre shape and become prone to haemolysis. In addition the sickled red cells block the capillaries to produce infarcts, particularly in the spleen and bones.

3. False
This disorder may be associated either with a hae-molysin or haemagglutinin, the antibody having maximum activity below body temperature, usually at about 20°C. Thus acute intravascular lysis occurs after exposure of the whole or part of the body to cold.

4. False
This is a rare chronic haemolytic disorder of insidious onset, most common in early middle life characterised by haemoglobinuria, weakness, fever and moderate splenomegaly. Intravascular haemolysis occurs mainly during sleep when a slight lowering of the pH occurs, lysis probably being caused by some of the red cells being abnormally sensitive to complement.

5. True
Thalassaemia major is the homozygous form of this disorder in which synthesis of the α or β chains of the haemoglobin molecule is defective. The condition often presents as an apparent haemolytic anaemia of infancy accompanied by pallor and splenomegaly, and the mean red cell survival time is grossly reduced.

17.3 The presence of Hb-A$_2$ ($\alpha_2 \lambda_2$) in the red corpuscles is associated with:

1. increased osmotic resistance of the red cells
2. reduced life span of the red corpuscles
3. congenital spherocytosis
4. thalassaemia
5. sickle-cell anaemia

1. True
Cells containing Hb-A$_2$ ($\alpha_2 \lambda_2$) are flatter than normal, compare this with spherocytosis. They are, therefore,

270

more resistant to haemolysis when incubated in a hypotonic solution.

2. True
The presence of abnormal haemoglobin in an erythrocyte reduces the life span of the erythrocyte from the normal of 100 to 120 days.

3. False
Congenital spherocytosis is associated with a membrane defect which causes the cell to be excessively permeable to sodium ions.

4. True
Thalassaemia is a disease associated with either a defect of the α or β polypeptide chains of the globin molecule. In the classic form the β chains are defective.

5. False
Sickle-cell anaemia is associated with Hb-S, Hb-S ($\alpha_2\beta_2^{6val}$) differing chemically from Hb-A in the substitution of valine for glutamic acid in the sixth position of the amino-acid sequence of the β chain.

17.4 Iron deficiency anaemia may be associated with the following:

1. A sensitive and painful glossitis
2. Dysphagia
3. A rise in the liver iron
4. Koilonychia
5. Chlorosis

1. False
A sensitive, painful glossitis is typical of vitamin B_{12} and folate deficiency although chronic iron deficiency leads to atrophy of the tongue papillae.

2. True
Dysphagia is a rare association with chronic iron deficiency. This combination is known as the Plummer–Vinson or Paterson–Kelly syndrome, a characteristic feature of which is the development of dysphagia due either to neuromuscular incoordination of the upper end of the oesophagus or the development of webs at the same level.

3. False
Demonstrable changes in iron metabolism develop before the Hb begins to fall. The first change is a depletion of the body stores of iron. This can be demonstrated either by liver biopsy or from specimens of aspirated bone marrow.

4. True
This is one of the characteristic features of severe iron deficiency anaemia. The nails of the radial fingers of the hand show the most pronounced changes; they become brittle and tend to split. Later they soften, become flatter and later even concave. Koilonychia is most marked in patients who immerse their hands in water.

5. True
This condition which is now no longer seen was first described in the sixteenth century. Chlorosis occurred in adolescent girls suffering from severe iron deficiency anaemia and was marked by the development of a yellowish or greenish complexion. The probable aetiology was a combination of a poor diet, rapid growth and the onset of menstruation.

17.5 The production of red blood cells is depressed by the following conditions:

1. Chronic renal failure
2. Excessive administration of glucocorticoids
3. Subacute rheumatic fever
4. Myxoedema
5. Disseminated breast cancer

1. True
Chronic renal failure is invariably associated with anaemia. This is believed to be due to marrow depression probably caused by the inadequate production of erythropoietin. The severity of the anaemia, however, does not always coincide with the degree of uraemia.

2. False
The administration of excessive quantities of glucocorticoids has little effect on erythropoiesis except indirectly as changes in the plasma volume occur.

However, in Cushing's disease a mild erythrocytosis may be present.

3. True
Anaemia is a common complication of subacute rheumatic fever in childhood particularly when the disease is accompanied by joint pains and active carditis.

4. True
In animals a normocytic, normochromic anaemia follows removal of the thyroid, the anaemia being corrected by the administration of thyroxine. In man the severity of the anaemia in myxoedema and its frequency vary according to the series examined. However, thyroid deficiency should always be considered in the differential diagnosis when a normocytic anaemia fails to respond to treatment.

5. True
Red cell production is depressed in disseminated breast cancer when the red marrow is replaced by malignant tissue.

17.6 Pathological destruction of red blood cells can take place in the following sites:

1. The submucosal plexus of the small intestine
2. The peripheral circulation
3. The liver
4. The spleen
5. The bone marrow

1. **False**
2. **True**
3. **True**
4. **True**
5. **True**

Pathological red cell destruction occurs in two major sites. Either within the peripheral circulation when the contents of the erythrocyte are liberated into the plasma or secondly, in intimate proximity to the cells of the mononuclear phagocyte system (3.4.5), a system previously known as the reticulo-endothelial system. In the latter sites the products of red cell destruction can be immediately phagocytosed.

Intravascular haemolysis can be caused by a number of factors which include:
  (a) Toxic substances such as lead, benzene and phenylhydrazine
  (b) Parasitic infections such as malaria
  (c) Invasive bacterial infections causing septicaemia
  (d) Following burns

Extravascular haemolysis is chiefly seen:
  (a) In the presence of structural abnormalities of the red cell, e.g. congenital spherocytosis and thalassaemia
  (b) When incomplete agglutinating antibodies are present in the circulation, e.g. in diffuse lupus erythematosus or ulcerative colitis
  (c) In the presence of diseases of the mononuclear-phagocyte system (reticuloendothelial system), e.g. Hodgkin's lymphoma

The submucosal plexus of the gastrointestinal tract plays no part in the destruction of red cells.

17.7 The commonest haemolytic disorder in the world is:

1. congenital spherocytosis
2. disseminated lupus erythematosus
3. malaria
4. G6PD deficiency
5. sickle disease

The correct answer is **3**. All the conditions listed cause haemolysis but malaria is the commonest of them all because of its widespread distribution. Haemolysis occurs in malaria due to parasitisation of the red cells by the merozoites which then go through further cycles of asexual proliferation until the red cell is destroyed. This occurs with every bout of fever.

17.8 The following haemolytic disorders are congenital:

1. Thalassaemia
2. March haemoglobinuria
3. Microangiopathic haemolytic anaemia
4. Ovalocytosis
5. G6PD deficiency

1. True
Thalassaemia is a complex disorder in which the main abnormality is a defect in the synthesis of one of the polypeptide chains of the globin of haemoglobin A. Heterozygotes show some evidence of mild haemolytic disease, thalassaemia minor, whereas homozygotes are severely affected and seldom survive beyond early adult life.

2. False
This condition of acute haemoglobinuria, usually mild, results from long marches. Haemolysis is believed to be caused by mechanical damage to the red cells as they flow through the plantar aspect of the feet during long marches on hard surfaces.

3. False
This condition is the result of disseminated intravascular coagulation and occurs in a variety of conditions including disseminated malignancy, fulminating septicaemia and the haemolytic uraemic syndrome. Severe haemolytic anaemia occurs associated with distortion and fragmentation of the red cells.

4. True
Ovalocytosis is a hereditary condition in which a high proportion of red cells are ovalocytes and many develop a rod-shaped deformity. The condition is transmitted as an autosomal dominant and the precise metabolic abnormality has yet to be established.

5. True
G6PD deficiency is a rare condition in which the life span of the red cells is shortened. G6PD is concerned with the maintenance of the NADP/NADPH ratio so that the majority of glutathione in the red cell is in the reduced state. How this substance maintains the integrity of the red cell membrane is unknown.

17.9 Congenital spherocytosis is a haemolytic disorder:

1. inherited as an autosomal recessive
2. associated with chronic anaemia
3. basically caused by a developmental defect of the red cell membrane

4. associated with massive enlargement of the spleen
5. in which the osmotic fragility of the red cell is diminished

1. False
Hereditary spherocytosis is inherited as an autosomal dominant of variable penetrance, the latter determining the clinical severity of the disease.

2. True
The majority of patients suffering from hereditary spherocytosis suffer from chronic anaemia, although some patients do not develop symptoms until adult life.

3. True
The fundamental defect in congenital spherocytosis is in the red cell membrane. This is unduly permeable to the passive influx of Na^+ ion. The accelerated metabolic activity necessary for the transport of Na^+ out of the cell is associated with increased ATPase activity, the breakdown of ATP and an increase in glycolysis and the turnover of membrane phospholipid. It is probably the loss of surface lipid which determines the critical change in shape of the red cell from that of a biconcave disc to a sphere.

4. False
This condition is associated with only moderate enlargement of the spleen. The spherocytes characteristic of this disease are trapped in the cords of Billroth.

5. False
Osmotic fragility is enhanced in congenital spherocytosis. It is this abnormality which led to the recognition of the disease towards the end of the nineteenth century.

17.10 Polycythaemia occurs in:

1. congenital cyanotic heart disease
2. tumours of the renal parenchyma, renal carcinoma
3. the carcinoid syndrome
4. lead poisoning
5. hypoxia

1. True
Intense polycythaemia is frequently present in congenital heart disease with the result that the blood volume is increased, primarily due to an increase in red cell volume. In consequence the haematocrit is high (see 5).

2. True
Polycythaemia occurs in association with renal carcinoma because of the high output of erythropoietin by some of these tumours.

3. False
The plethoric appearance of the face in the carcinoid syndrome which might suggest polycythaemia is due to telangiectasia of the skin together with release of the enzyme kallikrein from the tumour which produces bradykinin from plasma substrates.

4. False
Lead poisoning produces chronic anaemia which probably depends upon two factors:
  (a) Interference with synthesis of haemoglobin
  (b) Excessive fragility of the red cells

5. True
Hypoxia of any type, especially that associated with chronic respiratory insufficiency, congenital heart disease with right to left shunts, or living at high altitudes is a common cause of secondary polycythaemia. The bone marrow is stimulated by erythropoietin.

17.11 Megaloblastic anaemia may be caused by:

1. atrophy or ablation of the gastric mucosa
2. infestation with *Diphyllobothrium latum*
3. lesions involving the terminal ileum
4. over enthusiastic use of purgatives
5. small bowel blind loops

1. True
Atrophy of the gastric mucosa is the underlying cause of classic pernicious anaemia. Ablation of the gastric mucosa by total gastrectomy will lead to a megaloblastic anaemia after the natural reserves of B_{12} in the liver have been exhausted in about 3 to 4 years.

2. True

This helminth competes with the host for vitamin B_{12}. This type of megaloblastic anaemia is found only in Finland despite the world wide distribution of the worm.

3. True

The lesion may be inflammatory as in Crohn's disease or the bowel may have been resected. A megaloblastic anaemia follows because the terminal ileum is the site of absorption of vitamin B_{12} and folic acid.

4. False

Purgatives act on the colon which is not concerned with the absorption of vitamin B_{12} or folic acid.

5. True

Small bowel blind loops may be the result of a surgical procedure, e.g. jejunal resection followed by side to side or an end to side anastomosis. This causes a megaloblastic anaemia because the intrinsic factor–B_{12} complex normally formed in the stomach fails to reach its absorptive site in the distal ileum. This is due to the abnormal proliferation of bacteria in such loops which compete for and take up the IF-B_{12} complex. A similar situation may develop in patients suffering from jejunal diverticulosis.

17.12 The following abnormalities occur in pernicious anaemia:

1. A low haemoglobin
2. A decreased mean corpuscular haemoglobin (MCH)
3. An increased reticulocyte count
4. Antibodies to the parietal cells
5. A decrease in the circulating level of vitamin B_{12}

1. True

The definition of anaemia is a fall in the number of red cells or quantity of haemoglobin in a given volume of blood in the presence of a low or normal total blood volume. In pernicious anaemia the number of red cells is diminished but the plasma volume increases.

2. False

The mean corpuscular haemoglobin is elevated and

the mean corpuscular volume is greater than normal although individual cells show great variation in size.

3. False
It may be normal but rises rapidly once treatment begins. In percentage terms the reticulocyte count may rise within a week following a single intramuscular injection of vitamin B_{12} from 3 to 50.

4. True
Antibodies to both parietal cells and the intrinsic factor can be found in the majority of patients suffering from classical pernicious anaemia.

5. True
Vitamin B_{12}, the extrinsic factor, cannot be absorbed in the absence of the intrinsic factor (IF) which is produced by the parietal cells. Hence in classical pernicious anaemia the serum vitamin B_{12} is reduced.

17.13 In pernicious anaemia the following pathological changes may be seen:

1. Haemosiderosis
2. Atrophy of the gastric mucosa
3. A decrease in the volume of red marrow in the long bones
4. Extramedullary haemopoiesis
5. Demyelination of the lateral and dorsal columns, not associated with gliosis

1. True
Haemosiderin is ferritin with an iron content of about 36 per cent. This pigment forms brown insoluble granules which give the Prussian Blue reaction. Haemosiderosis occurs in pernicious anaemia because of haemolysis and the diversion of the iron normally present in the circulating haemoglobin to the tissues.

2. True
The mucosa of the stomach shows a generalised atrophic change with almost complete destruction of the specialised cells of the fundus including the parietal cells.

3. False

Increasing erythropoiesis leads to an extension of the red marrow.

4. True

In severe pernicious anaemia foci of ectopic erythropoiesis can be found in the liver and spleen.

5. True

This change, known as subacute combined degeneration, occurs only in pure vitamin B_{12} deficiency. It does not occur in folic acid deficiency.

17.14 The following biochemical changes occur in pernicious anaemia:

1. A raised serum vitamin B_{12}
2. A normal serum folate
3. A raised serum bilirubin
4. An increased alkaline phosphatase
5. A decreased plasma copper

1. False

The reverse is true, the serum vitamin B_{12} falls due to decreased absorption. This is caused by an absence of the intrinsic factor which is normally formed by the stomach. In pernicious anaemia a diffuse atrophic gastritis occurs.

2. True

In classical pernicious anaemia the serum folate levels are normal although the histidine test may produce abnormal FIGLU excretion.

3. True

In classical pernicious anaemia haemolysis occurs. This is sufficient to cause a slight elevation of the serum bilirubin, an increase in the amount of stercobilinogen in the faeces and moderate urobilinuria.

4. False

Alkaline phosphatase plays no part in the metabolism of haemoglobin.

5. False

Although copper is essential for normal erythropoiesis no changes occur in the concentration of this in the serum in pernicious anaemia.

17.15 An absolute lymphocytosis occurs in the following conditions:

1. Extensive skin diseases such as psoriasis, eczema, pemphigus
2. Löeffler's syndrome
3. Tuberculosis
4. Pertussis
5. Chronic lymphatic leukaemia

1. False
Chronic and extensive skin diseases such as those named in the question are not associated with a lymphocytosis.

2. False
Löeffler's syndrome is a pulmonary eosinophilia which is associated with a hypersensitivity state in which the commonest allergen is a worm such as *Ascaris lumbricoides*. Many other factors have been implicated including several drugs such as para-aminosalicylic acid and chlorpropamide. An eosinophilia occurs but this is not associated with a lymphocytosis. Clinically a cough develops and transient areas of infiltration may be seen in plain radiographs of the chest.

3. True
Chronic infections such as tuberculosis and syphilis may be accompanied by an absolute lymphocytosis.

4. True
Whooping cough is accompanied by a marked lymphocytosis even before the classical whoop has developed, counts as high as 100 000 per μl may be found.

5. True
In chronic lymphatic leukaemia the absolute lymphocyte count may exceed 100 000 per μl. The majority of cells appear to be normal mature small lymphocytes but larger more primitive cells are also found. In many cases the leukaemic lymphocytes possess surface immunoglobulins characteristic of B-cells.

17.16 Acute myeloblastic leukaemia:

1. is most common in young adults

2. is associated with the presence of a large number of primitive cells in the marrow and peripheral blood
3. is associated with peripheral white counts in excess of 100 000 per μl
4. may be associated with a normal white count
5. marrow aspirates show decreased cellularity

1. False
The highest incidence of any form of leukaemia occurs in the first 5 years of life and in the fifth decade, but overall before puberty acute lymphoblastic is commoner than acute myeloblastic leukaemia.

2. True
In acute leukaemia the predominant cell in the marrow or blood is the myeloblast, lymphoblast or monoblast according to the type of leukaemia.

3. False
In acute leukaemia the total white count is only moderately raised, counts between 20 000 and 50 000 per μl being common. In contrast in the various forms of chronic leukaemia the peripheral white count may exceed 300 000 per μl.

4. True
In over one-third of all cases the total white count is normal or even reduced, so-called aleukaemic leukaemia. However, even in these cases primitive cells can almost always be found in the peripheral blood.

5. False
The typical picture in acute leukaemia is an increase in cellularity. Sections of the marrow show replacement of the fat spaces by primitive leukaemic cells.

17.17 Myeloid metaplasia may be associated with:

1. a variable peripheral white count
2. extramedullary haemopoiesis
3. the Philadelphia chromosome
4. a decreased number of megakaryocytes in the marrow
5. anaemia

1. True
The white cell count in the peripheral blood may range from 3000 to 30 000 per μl.

2. True
The term myeloid metaplasia is used to describe extramedullary haemopoiesis which occurs chiefly in the spleen and liver and only rarely in other organs.

3. False
The Philadelphia chromosome, a deletion of the long arms of one of the chromosome 22 pair in the white cell, is found in 90 per cent of sufferers from chronic myeloid leukaemia. It is not found in myeloid metaplasia.

4. False
One of the characteristic features of myeloid metaplasia is the presence of an increased number of megakaryocytes in the bone marrow.

5. True
Myeloid metaplasia may be associated with either anaemia or polycythaemia, the former is occasionally sufficiently severe to require blood transfusion.

17.18 Chronic myeloid leukaemia is associated with:

1. the presence of large numbers of myeloblasts in the peripheral blood
2. a very variable total white count
3. massive splenomegaly
4. lymph nodes enlargement
5. hepatomegaly

1. False
The dominant white cell in the peripheral circulation is the neutrophil myelocyte and only a few myeloblasts are present.

2. True
The white count may vary between 15 000 and 500 000 per μl. Sufficient mature cells are usually present to make the diagnosis without difficulty.

3. True
Massive splenomegaly occurs because this organ becomes infiltrated by myelocytes and polymorphonuclear leucocytes. Pale infarcts are common.

283

4. False

In chronic myeloid leukaemia the lymph nodes are usually normal in size in contrast to the situation in chronic lymphatic leukaemia in which the lymph nodes are usually enlarged early in the course of the disease.

5. True

In chronic myeloid leukaemia primitive cells are found in the sinusoids. In contrast in chronic lymphocytic leukaemia the primitive cells infiltrate the periportal areas.

17.19 Chronic myeloid leukaemia differs from chronic lymphatic leukaemia in that:

1. in the former the predominant white cell in the circulation is the leucocyte
2. the total white count is higher in chronic lymphatic leukaemia
3. in the former the proliferating marrow cells possess the Philadelphia chromosome
4. the latter is more common in an older age group than is the former
5. the former disease tends to develop into a more aggressive type of acute leukaemia

1. True

The blood picture in chronic myeloid leukaemia is dominated by the presence of myelocytes, polymorphonuclear leucocytes and intermediate forms.

2. False

The total white count is highest in chronic myeloid leukaemia reaching 300 000 per μl as compared to 100 000 per μl in the latter.

3. True

The Philadelphia chromosome is an abnormal 22 chromosome present in the white and red blood cell precursors in the marrow in chronic myeloid leukaemia.

4. False

Both diseases are commoner in middle and later life although chronic myeloid leukaemia occasionally occurs in younger individuals.

5. True
Many patients who have suffered from chronic myeloid leukaemia may enter a terminal phase in which
acute leukaemia develops. This is associated with
anaemia, infection and thrombocytopenic bleeding.

**17.20 Chronic lymphocytic leukaemia is associated
with:**

1. a marked increase in the number of lymphocytes
   in the peripheral blood
2. the early appearance of anaemia
3. an early bleeding tendency
4. an increase in the serum globulin concentration
5. an increase in the number of B-lymphocytes in the
   blood

1. True
The number of white cells in chronic lymphocytic
leukaemia may reach 100 000 per μl. The majority of
these are lymphocytes, with the appearance of normal mature small lymphocytes. A small proportion,
however, are larger, more primitive cells.

2. False
Since the disease originates in the lymphoid tissues
extensive replacement of the haemopoietic marrow
occurs late. Hence anaemia is a terminal manifesta-
tion of the disease.

3. False
For the same reason that 2 is false, although in some
patients a mild thrombocytopenia may occur in the
course of the disease, possibly of autoimmune
nature.

4. False
Since extensive involvement of the lymphoid tissues
occurs relatively early a reduction in the normal
plasma immunoglobulins occurs associated with a
decreased resistance to bacterial infection.

5. True
In the majority of cases the predominant lymphocyte
is the B-cell although occasional cases occur which
appear to be of T-cell type.

17.21 Monocytic leukaemia:

1. is the commonest form of leukaemia
2. is associated with monocytes or monoblasts in the peripheral blood
3. may present with increasing anaemia
4. is associated with nodular infiltrative skin lesions
5. can present as an acute myelo-monocytic form

1. False
Monocytic leukaemia is a relatively uncommon form of leukaemia. It accounts for less than 10 per cent of all the leukaemias although it accounts for approximately 20 per cent of acute leukaemias.

2. True
The total white count may be relatively low although it may reach 250 000 per μl, the majority of cells being monocytes or monoblasts. These may exhibit pseudopodial cytoplasmic projections, a fine peripheral cytoplasmic PAS+ve granularity and lysozyme production.

3. True
This is a characteristic feature, however, of all types of leukaemia. Severe anaemia may arise so suddenly that the individual is prostrated with weakness.

4. True
This is one of the characteristic features of this type of leukaemia, the skin being infiltrated by monocytes or monoblasts.

5. True
This is the Naegeli type of leukaemia in which an admixture of myeloid cells and monoblasts appear, presumably due to the progenitor cell being able to differentiate into either type of cell line.

17.22 An enlarged lymph node which is excised is found by histological examination to be packed with tubercles consisting of epithelioid cells and giant cells. The tuberculin and Heaf test are negative. Which of the following diseases should then be considered as the probable cause of the lymphadenopathy:

1. Hodgkin's disease
2. Tuberculosis

3. Sarcoidosis
4. Syphilis
5. Toxoplasmosis

1. False
Hodgkin's disease is not associated with follicle formation or epithelioid cells although giant cells, known as the Reed–Sternberg cells, do appear.

2. False
If the node was tuberculous either the tuberculin or Heaf test should be positive.

3. True
This is the classic picture of a node affected by sarcoidosis. The giant cells of sarcoidosis resemble foreign body giant cells rather than the Langhans cells characteristic of tuberculosis. A further pathological difference is that caseation does not occur in the centre of the follicles. The diagnosis can be confirmed by the presence of a positive Kveim Test.

4. False
In 'secondary syphilis' a generalised enlargement of the lymph nodes occurs in some 2 to 3 months after exposure. Affected nodes show an increased number of plasma cells and macrophages and specific investigations such as the Wassermann reaction would be necessary to confirm the diagnosis.

5. False
The chief histological features of lymph nodes affected by toxoplasmosis are the presence of large cells, probably macrophages, scattered singly or in small groups throughout both the cortex and medulla. The sinuses are filled with smaller cells of uncertain nature. Toxoplasmosis is due to infection with the protozoon, *Toxoplasma gondii*.

17.23 Hodgkin's lymphoma has recently been re-classified into four histological groups. Regardless of classification, however, which of the following cell types are found in the lymph nodes in this disease?

1. Lymphocytes
2. Basophils
3. Eosinophils
4. Reed–Sternberg cells
5. Polymorphonuclear leucocytes

1. True

In all forms of Hodgkin's disease these cells are found in the lymph nodes. They are, however, most commonly found in the lymphocytic predominant type of the disease (Rye Classification).

2. False

Basophilic white cells are not found in the lymph nodes in any type of Hodgkin's disease.

3. True

Eosinophils are found particularly in the lymphocyte predominant and the nodular sclerotic types (Rye Classification).

4. True

These cells were described by Reed in 1902 and by Sternberg in 1898 and are usually known as Reed–Sternberg cells despite the fact that the same cell had already been described some years previously by Greenfield of Edinburgh in 1878. The Reed–Sternberg cell is a giant cell in which the nucleus is bifid or bilobed, the two halves being virtually identical. When more than two nuclei are present they are usually arranged in a horse shoe fashion or piled one on top of another. These are the typical cells of Hodgkin's disease and are present in all varieties of the disease although commonest in 'mixed cellularity' type of disease.

5. True

Polymorphonuclear leucocytes are found either diffusely infiltrating affected lymph nodes or in marked aggregations suggesting the presence of micro-abscesses in the nodes.

17.24 The chief characteristics of Burkitt's lymphoma are:

1. that it is commonest in young adults
2. it is associated with the Epstein Barr virus
3. it is uncommon in malarial areas
4. the commonest parts of the body involved are the facial bones and lower jaw
5. the characteristic cells of the tumour are poorly differentiated large lymphocytes and large pale histocytes

1. False
This condition is commonest in children in East and Central Africa.

2. True
It is associated with the virus although it is doubtful whether this is the chief aetiological factor.

3. False
The commonest areas in which the disease is found are the malarial areas although it occasionally occurs elsewhere. This association with malaria suggests that an infective oncogenic agent transmitted by insects plays a role in the aetiology.

4. True
In approximately 50 per cent of all cases either the upper or lower jaws are involved and the teeth become loosened as the bones expand. Other regions involved are the lymph nodes of the abdomen, although the liver and spleen are rarely diseased.

5. True
The histological picture of Burkitt's lymphoma is often described as resembling a 'starry sky'. It is similar to that seen in the secondary germinal centres of lymph nodes undergoing a reactive hyperplasia.

17.25 The plasma prothrombin time is increased:

1. in hepatocellular disease
2. in obstructive jaundice
3. in haemophilia
4. in Christmas disease
5. following splenectomy

1. True
Severe hepatocellular disease is incompatible with the normal synthesis of prothrombin and as a result the prothrombin time is prolonged.

2. True
In obstructive jaundice a decrease in prothrombin concentration occurs because obstruction of the biliary tree prevents bile salts entering the gut. As a result the fat soluble vitamin K, which is essential for prothrombin formation, fails to be absorbed.

3. False
This disease, although associated with bleeding, is due to the absence of the procoagulant activity of Factor VIII. The prothrombin time is normal.

4. False
This condition, first recognised in 1952, is due to a congenital absence of Factor IX. The prothrombin time is normal.

5. False
Splenectomy does not affect the prothrombin time but may be associated with a temporary thrombocythaemia. This may cause post-operative thrombotic episodes to occur.

17.26 Disorders of clotting occur in association with:

1. vitamin A deficiency
2. vitamin K deficiency
3. hereditary angioneurotic oedema
4. haemophilia
5. obstructive jaundice

1. False
Vitamin A plays no part in the clotting mechanisms but is concerned with the maintenance of the normal structure and function of epithelial tissues. Avitaminosis A results in squamous metaplasia in a number of epithelial tissues and in addition night blindness due to a deficiency of rhodopsin pigment in the retina.

2. True
Vitamin K is necessary for the hepatic synthesis of prothrombin and clotting factors VII, IX and X. Because of this the prothrombin time is increased in the presence of a vitamin K deficiency. Vitamin K deficiency accompanies many of the malabsorption syndromes.

3. False
Hereditary angioneurotic oedema is due to the absence of C1 esterase inhibitor which inhibits the action of Hageman factor. This defect causes an increase in the amount of kallikrein and an increased production of kinin. No direct effect on the clotting cascade occurs.

4. True
Haemophilia is a hereditary condition due to a sex linked recessive deficiency of antihaemophilic globulin or clotting Factor VIII. This results in a severe bleeding diathesis, bleeding being most commonly precipitated by trauma and involving the muscles and joints rather than the mucous membranes and the skin.

5. True
Both vitamin K deficiency and hypoprothrombinaemia occur in obstructive jaundice due to the exclusion of bile salts from the intestine which results in an inability to absorb fat soluble vitamins.

17.27 The formation of a clot is affected by the following substances:

1. Zinc
2. Calcium
3. Factor B
4. Factor IX
5. Kallikrein

1. False
Zinc plays no role in clotting but is probably of some importance in wound healing.

2. True
Calcium ions are necessary for all phases of the clotting cascade.

3. False
Factor B plays no part in the clotting of blood. Factor B or C3 proactivator plays an important role in the alternative pathway of complement activation.

4. True
Factor IX or Christmas factor is part of the intrinsic clotting pathway. Deficiency of Factor IX occurs as a rare sex linked recessive trait producing a bleeding disorder similar to haemophilia.

5. False
Kallikrein, which is chiefly produced by the basophil white cells, is the enzyme which converts kininogen to kinin. It plays no part in the clotting of blood. The kinins produced by its action are important in

anaphylaxis in which condition there is vasodilatation associated with increased vascular permeability.

17.28 Haemorrhagic lesions may occur as a result of:

1. vitamin B deficiency
2. vitamin C deficiency
3. retinol deficiency
4. the nephrotic syndrome
5. penicillin therapy

1. False
Vitamin B deficiency is not associated with haemorrhagic lesions. Classically thiamine deficiency causes beri-beri; riboflavine deficiency, angular stomatitis and glossitis and nicotinic acid deficiency pellagra which is associated with dermatitis, diarrhoea and dementia.

2. True
Vitamin C (ascorbic acid) is important in the production of collagen and in the synthesis of intercellular cement of the vascular endothelium. Avitaminosis C causes one of the classical deficiency diseases, i.e. scurvy, one of the manifestations of which is the appearance of haemorrhagic lesions particularly involving the gums and skin around the base of the hair follicles.

3. False
Retinol is vitamin A, deficiency of this vitamin does not cause haemorrhagic lesions. It causes night blindness followed by xerophthalmia and keratomalacia.

4. False
There is no tendency to develop haemorrhagic lesions in the nephrotic syndrome which is associated with widespread subcutaneous oedema due to loss of protein in the urine.

5. True
Procaine penicillin is one of a group of drugs including aspirin, phenacetin and the sulphonamides which may give rise to petechial haemorrhages in the skin. The basis of the phenomenon may be immune complex related to the Arthus phenomenon and in a number of other situations including aspirin

idiosyncrasy, an allergic reaction cannot be excluded.

17.29 Disseminated intravascular coagulation is a complication of:

1. surgical operations such as prostatectomy or open heart surgery
2. malignant disease
3. thrombocythaemia
4. the overadministration of thrombokinase
5. endotoxaemic shock

1. True
One theory advanced to explain the development of this condition in post-operative patients is that particulate matter such as fibres of collagen released from injured blood vessels induces platelet aggregation. The liberation of adenosine diphosphate (ADP) from affected platelets then leads to further platelet aggregation.

2. True
Patients suffering from malignant disease of the prostate, bronchus, pancreas and stomach are particularly liable to this complication.

3. True
Any condition which leads to an increase in the number of platelets in the blood such as polycythaemia vera or splenectomy may be followed by thrombosis in small blood vessels.

4. False
Thrombokinase is used in the treatment of patients in whom intravascular thrombosis and coagulation has occurred. It has been used for example in patients who have suffered from a pulmonary embolus.

5. True
Endotoxaemic shock caused by the endotoxins of Gram negative organisms induces platelet aggregation and hence the deposition of intravascular fibrin. This then stimulates fibrinolysis. If coagulation continues the clotting factors are depleted with the result that afibrinogenaemia follows leading finally to uncontrolled bleeding.

17.30 The following functions are carried out by platelets:

1. Binding of antigen-antibody complexes
2. Secretion of clotting factors
3. Secretion of prostaglandins
4. Release of the Hageman factor
5. Release of vasoactive amines

1. True
Antigen-antibody complexes activate complement and are bound to platelets by a process known as immune adherence through a receptor for C3b.

2. False
Although platelets play a vital role in haemostasis they do not release any of the factors concerned in either the intrinsic or extrinsic clotting pathways. Plasma contains all the factors necessary for clotting to take place after contact activation or tissue damage. Platelet factor 3 is an altered state of the surface of the platelets and not a secretion.

3. True
Platelets release prostaglandin E_2. This is concerned with the release of ADP, a substance which causes the platelets to adhere together. E type prostaglandins are also proinflammatory agents, acting via cyclic AMP.

4. False
The Hageman factor (Factor XII) is a plasma protein which migrates on electrophoresis as a β or γ globulin. It is activated by contact and this is the first step in the intrinsic clotting pathway.

5. True
Platelets release 5-hydroxytryptamine (serotonin) which is a potent vasoactive material causing vasodilatation and an increase in capillary permeability.

17.31 Thrombocytopenia can be caused by:

1. deficiency of clotting factors
2. haemorrhage
3. diuretics
4. measles virus
5. telangiectasia

1. False
A deficiency of clotting factors causes bleeding diseases such as haemophilia and Christmas disease, but there is no reduction in platelet numbers in either of these conditions. Thrombocytopenia is, however, associated with a bleeding diathesis, because platelets are necessary for haemostasis. Platelets seal small vessels, which are injured, by adhering to their surface, catalysing the intrinsic clotting system through surface lipoprotein.

2. True
Severe haemorrhage or repeated bleeding may cause thrombocytopenia. This loss, if severe, must be made good by the transfusion of fresh blood. Stored blood does not contain viable platelets and is, therefore, useless.

3. True
The thiazide diuretics are among the many drugs which can give rise to a thrombocytopenia. This is considered to be produced immunologically by the binding of the drug to the platelets. Antibody is then being formed against the drug which acts as a hapten.

4. True
Viruses, such as the measles virus, may impair platelet production by colonising the parent megakaryocytes. Others may actually destroy platelets or form immune complexes binding to the platelets leading to their destruction.

5. False
Hereditary haemorrhagic telangiectasia may be the cause of haemorrhages due to the associated vascular defect even though the concentration of clotting factors and the number of platelets is normal.

17.32 Thrombocytopenia:

1. may occur as an autoimmune phenomenon
2. is caused by sulphonamides
3. is associated with an increased bleeding time
4. is associated with an increased clotting time
5. the thromboplastin generation test is useful in its recognition

1. True

Idiopathic thrombocytopenic purpura is associated with IgG autoantibodies against platelets. A similar type of thrombocytopenia may occur in other recognised autoimmune diseases such as systemic lupus erythematosus.

2. True

Sulphonamides, thiazide diuretics, quinidine and stibophen, are among the drugs that give rise to thrombocytopenia. The drug that has been most extensively investigated is Sedormid. In Sedormid purpura this drug acts as a hapten, which binds to the serum proteins with the result that antibody formation occurs. Antigen-antibody complexes then bind to the platelets resulting in their destruction.

3. True

The bleeding time, normally between one and nine minutes, is the time taken for a small puncture to stop bleeding. The duration of the bleeding time is dependent upon normal platelet activity and thrombocytopenia, therefore, from whatever cause, will cause a prolonged bleeding time.

4. False

This is the time taken for blood to clot in a test tube and normally takes between 5 and 15 minutes. An increase in the clotting time occurs when there is a deficiency of clotting factors as in haemophilia whereas in thrombocytopenia the clotting time is normal.

5. False

The thromboplastin generation test is a complex test which is used to identify particular defects in the clotting factors in the serum. In the first stage thromboplastin (prothrombinase) is generated using a mixture of serum, kaolin absorbed plasma, platelets and calcium. The thromboplastin is then assayed by adding the mixture to normal plasma. This test will not help in the diagnosis of thrombocytopenia, although it is extremely valuable in pointing to the precise defect in the clotting factors.

17.33 Platelets contribute to haemostasis by liberating:

1. 5-hydroxytryptamine (serotonin)

2. phospholipids
3. plasminogen
4. bradykinin
5. calcitonin

1. True
5-hydroxytryptamine liberated from the platelets is a vasoconstrictor augmenting the normal vascular contraction which follows injury.

2. True
Platelet phospholipid and calcium is essential to the intrinsic coagulation system.

3. False
Plasminogen is the inactive precursor of plasmin which is carried in the plasma. Whenever fibrinogen is laid down it carries with it sufficient plasminogen to ensure its subsequent lysis.

4. False
Bradykinin is a powerful vasodilator probably derived from an α_2-globulin in the plasma by the action of the enzyme kallikrein.

5. False
This hormone is derived from the parafollicular (C) cells of the thyroid and is one of three important factors concerned in the regulation of plasma calcium concentration, the other factors being parathyroid hormone and vitamin D_3. It has no effect on haemostasis.

17.34 Thrombocytopenic purpura differs from non-thrombocytopenic purpura in that:

1. in the former condition the platelet count is reduced
2. in the latter the main defect is in the capillaries
3. the former may follow systemic disease
4. the latter may result from allergy
5. petechiae occur in the former but not in the latter

1. True
When the platelet count is reduced below 150 000 per μl thrombocytopenia is present. Abnormal bleeding is uncommon, however, if the platelet count remains higher than 60 000 per μl.

2. True
Platelets are normally involved in preventing bleeding from normal capillaries. When the platelet count is normal but the capillaries are abnormal, e.g. due to the action of endotoxins, bleeding occurs.

3. True
Among the many causes of thrombocytopenic purpura are systemic lupus erythematosus and chronic lymphatic leukaemia.

4. True
The classical example of non-thrombocytopenic purpura is Henoch–Schönlein purpura, otherwise known as anaphylactoid purpura. This condition commonly develops some two to three weeks after a streptococcal upper respiratory infection.

5. False
In both types of purpura small haemorrhages occur from capillaries throughout the body causing petechiae in the skin, mucous membranes and serous surfaces. Bleeding into the mucous membrane of the gastrointestinal tract produces abdominal colic, bleeding in the urinary tract produces haematuria.

17.35 Consecutive clot:

1. occurs in arteries distal to a thrombotic obstruction
2. occurs in the collateral branches of an artery following obstruction to the main vessel
3. occurs in veins after the cessation of blood flow
4. extends proximally to the entrance of the next venous tributary
5. is formed of coralline thrombus

1. False
Consecutive clot occurs only in veins.

2. False
For the above reason.

3. True
When the blood flow in a vein has come to a halt the process of thrombosis ceases and clotting follows. A consecutive clot develops proximal to that point at

which stagnation becomes complete. Normally the clot extends proximally to the entrance of the next venous tributary. At this point the tip of the clot may become invaded by granulation tissue from the wall of the vessel in which the clot is occurring and its surface may become covered with endothelium. By this means propagation of the clot is halted. Alternatively clotting may continue proximally over a considerable distance leading to the clinical syndromes of phlegmasia alba or caerulea dolens.

4. True
As stated above.

5. False
Coralline thrombus occurs in veins in which the blood is still flowing. This type of thrombus is so named because it is composed of alternating layers of fused platelets and fibrin, the latter containing entrapped red cells. This configuration is best seen on longitudinal sections through the centre of the thrombus. Retraction of the fibrin causes a ripple effect and the elevated platelet ridges between the fibrin form the so-called lines of Zahn.

Section 18. ENDOCRINOLOGY

18.1 Phaeochromocytoma may be associated with:

1. paroxysmal hypertension
2. sweating
3. neurofibromatosis
4. a fall in blood pressure on palpating the abdomen
5. paroxysmal hypotension

1. True
Paroxysmal hypertension usually occurs early in the disease when noradrenaline is being intermittently released. Commonly, however, by the time a clinical diagnosis is reached a sustained hypertension is present due to constant outpouring of catechol amines.

2. True
This symptom, also due to the overproduction of catechol amines, may be paroxysmal or continuous.

3. True
Neurofibromatosis occurs in association with phaeochromocytoma in 5 per cent of all patients.

4. False
In approximately 50 per cent of patients suffering from phaeochromocytoma palpating the abdomen on the side of the tumour leads to a rise in blood pressure.

5. True
The possible explanation for this phenomenon is that an increase in the concentration of circulating catechol amines leads to a decrease in plasma and total blood volume.

18.2 Increased amounts of erythropoietin are found in the plasma:

1. in pernicious anaemia
2. in iron deficiency anaemia
3. following bleeding
4. in erythroblastosis foetalis
5. in Kwashiorkor

1. True
2. True
3. True
4. True
5. False

Erythropoietin is a glycoprotein which can be inactivated by mild acid hydrolysis or by inducing the formation of antibodies. Its production is regulated by an exquisitely sensitive feed back mechanism and in man only a relatively minor bleed is necessary to produce a rapid increase in the plasma concentration.

Erythropoietin may be formed in the kidney. An alternative hypothesis has, however, been advanced suggesting that the kidney produces a renal erythropoietin factor (REF). This then behaves like an enzyme acting upon a substrate in the plasma.

Erythropoietin probably acts directly on the primitive stem cell to stimulate normal red cell differentiation.

Increased amounts are found in the plasma in all conditions listed above with the exception of kwashiorkor.

18.3 An eosinophil adenoma of the anterior hypophysis is associated with:

1. enlargement of the sella turcica
2. hypertrophy and hyperplasia of the soft tissues throughout the body
3. excessive growth of the acral parts
4. premature closure of the epiphyses
5. impaired glucose tolerance

1. True
Eosinophil adenomata commonly grow to such a size that the sella turcica is enlarged, this being usually demonstrated by radiological examination. In addition enlargement of the gland causes pressure on the optic chiasma which eventually causes visual impairment in over half the cases.

2. True
Hyperplasia and hypertrophy occur because the secretion of somatotrophin (growth hormone) is excessive in this type of tumour. Should, however, the tumour undergo cystic degeneration or infarction the progressive development of gigantism or acromegaly ceases.

3. True
This is the change which gives rise to the name 'acromegaly'. Acromegaly occurs when the excessive somatotrophin excretion begins following fusion of the epiphyses and, therefore, only about 40 per cent of acromegalic patients gain in height. In the majority of sufferers the hands become 'spade-like' due to an overgrowth of the soft tissues and cortical thickening of the phalangeal bones, together with 'tufting' of the distal phalanges.

4. False
Fusion of the epiphyses occurs normally. However, the time at which somatotrophin overproduction begins is important. If oversecretion begins prior to fusion of the epiphyses gigantism develops with the long bones participating in proportionate growth whereas if oversecretion begins after epiphyseal fusion little increase in height normally occurs and the classic acromegalic is produced.

5. True
Impaired glucose tolerance occurs in about 50 per cent of patients and clinical diabetes in about 10 per cent.

18.4 Primary thyrotoxicosis is always accompanied by:

1. increased iodine uptake by the gland
2. a raised protein bound iodine
3. exophthalmos
4. hypercalcaemia
5. pernicious anaemia

1. True

Except in T_3 thyrotoxicosis hyperthyroidism is almost invariably associated with an increased uptake of iodine. Uptake is also increased in disorders in which accumulated iodine is inefficiently or ineffectively used to synthesise and secrete active hormone.

2. True

This test was once the mainstay of thyroid diagnosis but is now seldom used. The serum PBI measures the following:

(a) The iodine in T_4
(b) The small quantities of iodine in T_3
(c) A great variety of iodinated materials of exogenous origin that are bound to protein and a class of compounds, usually of endogenous origin, termed iodoproteins in which iodine is covalently bound within the peptide sequence of the protein molecule. The latter are commonly found in the sera of patients with Hashimoto's disease.

3. False

Exophthalmos is not necessarily present in patients suffering from primary thyrotoxicosis. The mechanism by which exophthalmos is produced remains to be elucidated. There is no doubt, however, that the anatomical deformity is caused by the deposition of mucopolysaccharides in the retro-orbital fat and the extrinsic muscles of the eye. In the majority of patients suffering from exophthalmos the plasma contains raised levels of LATS which is a gamma-globulin distinct from TSH.

4. True

Thyrotoxicosis is associated with increased excretion of calcium and phosphorus in the urine and stool. In some patients this may be so great that bone density is reduced and pathological fractures occur.

5. False
Approximately 3 per cent of patients with primary thyrotoxicosis have pernicious anaemia and a further 3 per cent have intrinsic factor auto-antibody together with a normal absorption of vitamin B_{12}.

18.5 Abnormal aggregation of lymphocytes occurs in the thyroid in the following pathological conditions:

1. Follicular carcinoma
2. Medullary carcinoma
3. Lymphadenoid goitre
4. Reidel's struma
5. Primary thyrotoxicosis

1. False
An excessive lymphocytic infiltration does not occur in this condition which is one of the two well differentiated forms of malignant disease of the thyroid. Some areas of such a tumour bear a close resemblance to normal thyroid tissue although the follicles generally are smaller and contain lesser amounts of colloid but in other areas the tumour is composed of solid sheets of cells.

2. False
Medullary tumours comprise only 5 to 10 per cent of thyroid neoplasms. They consist of cells with widely varying morphological features and arrangements in which papillary folds or follicles do not occur. An abundant hyaline stroma is present which has the staining properties of amyloid.

3. True
Lymphocytic infiltration is the characteristic feature of lymphadenoid goitre (Hashimoto's disease). In the majority of cases histological examination of the gland also reveals the destruction of the follicular cells and degeneration and fragmentation of the surrounding basement membrane. The interstitial tissue is infiltrated with lymphocytes and typical lymphoid follicles with germinal centres may be seen.

4. False
In Riedel's thyroiditis the thyroid undergoes a fibrotic change which extends into the adjacent struc-

303

tures. This change may be associated with abnormal fibrosis elsewhere in the body especially in the posterior mediastinum, producing superior mediastinal obstruction and in the retroperitoneal tissues causing the development of bilateral hydronephrosis and eventually renal failure.

5. True
The characteristic histopathological picture of primary thyrotoxicosis is one in which the follicles are small and lined by hyperplastic columnar epithelium with in addition varying degrees of lymphocytic infiltration which may form lymphoid follicles.

18.6 Primary hyperparathyroidism is associated with:

1. bone cysts
2. carcinoma of the parathyroid glands
3. dystrophic calcification
4. hypertension
5. anorexia

1. True
Histological examination of the bones in primary hyperparathyroidism shows generalised osteitis fibrosa. An increased formation and resorption of bone is evident and excessive numbers of osteoclasts can be seen on the trabeculae.

2. True
Carcinoma is the rarest parathyroid pathology causing primary hyperparathyroidism. A malignant tumour of a solitary gland accounting for only approximately 2 per cent of all cases. Clinically, malignancy should be suspected if a mass is palpable in the neck.

3. False
Dystrophic calcification only occurs in degenerate tissues. In primary hyperparathyroidism the accompanying hypercalcaemia is followed by calcification in normal tissues such as the kidney, metastatic calcification, which leads to nephrocalcinosis.

4. True
Hypertension occurs in primary hyperparathyroidism when the degree of renal damage produced by

the development of nephrocalcinosis has become severe enough to impair renal function.

5. True
The anorexia accompanying primary hyperparathyroidism may be due to one of three causes:
    (a) The hypercalcaemia alone
    (b) The presence of a co-existing duodenal ulcer
    (c) Recurrent pancreatitis

18.7 The plasma acid phosphatase concentration increases in:

1. Paget's disease (osteitis deformans)
2. idiopathic hypercalciuria
3. prostatic cancer
4. medullary carcinoma of the thyroid
5. rickets

1. False
Osteitis deformans is associated with an elevation of the alkaline phosphatase, the acid phosphatase is unaffected.

2. False
Idiopathic hypercalciuria is not associated with any change in the acid phosphatase levels. The high renal calcium output in this condition is possibly caused by the excessive intestinal absorption of this cation by an increase in vitamin-D-like or $1,25 \, (OH)_2 \, D_3$ activity.

3. True
In prostatic cancer the acid phosphatase rises above the normal level of 0 to 4 KA units/100 ml. High values occur particularly when the disease is disseminated because both normal and malignant prostatic epithelium secrete large quantities of this enzyme.

4. False
The only significant biochemical abnormality associated with medullary tumours of the thyroid is the hypersecretion of calcitonin.

5. False
Classical rickets is caused by a deficient intake of vitamin D in infancy. An increase in the concentra-

tion of alkaline phosphatase occurs without any change in the acid phosphatase.

18.8 The Zollinger-Ellison syndrome is associated with:

1. β-cell tumours of the pancreas
2. chronic duodenal ulceration
3. cholereiform diarrhoea
4. parathyroid adenomata
5. phaeochromocytoma

1. False
This syndrome is caused by non-β-cell islet cell tumours which in approximately two thirds of patients are malignant. This is clinically important since the surgeon is forced to direct his attention to the target organ, i.e. the stomach, leaving the tumour itself *in situ*.

2. True
The stomach is maximally stimulated by the presence of the gastrin secreting tumour and chronic duodenal ulceration follows. These ulcers may be multiple and even occur in the descending part of the duodenum or upper jejunum.

3. True
The gastric acid is normally neutralised by the alkaline pancreatic juices but the large quantities secreted in this syndrome cannot be neutralised by this means. Thus excessive quantities of acid reach the small bowel causing an acid enteritis associated with exceedingly fluid stools. An additional factor is probably the direct hormonal effect of gastrin on the transport of fluid and electrolytes.

4. True
Islet cell tumours producing gastrin are sometimes associated with parathyroid and pituitary adenomata. This particular 'cluster' is known as multiple endocrine adenoma, Type I.

5. False
Phaeochromocytoma are not associated with the Zollinger–Ellison syndrome but with medullary carcinoma of the thyroid and less frequently parathyroid adenomata.

18.9 The following tumours of the ovary secrete hormones:

1. Arrhenoblastoma
2. Dysgerminoma
3. Dermoid cysts
4. Papillary cystadenoma
5. Granulosa-theca cell tumour

1. True
These tumours account for less than 1 per cent of all solid ovarian tumours which secrete androgens with the result that masculinisation takes place in affected women. Seventy per cent occur below the age of forty.

2. True
Some, but not all, dysgerminomas secrete androgens and are, therefore, associated with the development of virilism.

3. True
Dermoid cysts may contain foci of chromaffin tissue which secrete serotonin. Rarer still are cysts consisting almost exclusively of thyroid tissue, the struma ovarii, which are sufficiently differentiated to produce thyroxine.

4. False
Papillary cystadenoma is one of the commoner tumours of the ovary. They are frequently bilateral, commonly reaching 10 cm in diameter. They may consist of a single main cyst on the inner surface of which are multiple papilliform projections. The contents are usually clear fluid unless complications such as torsion have occurred.

5. True
This tumour accounts for between 15 and 20 per cent of all solid ovarian neoplasms. Producing oestrogens they commonly present with polymenorrhoea but they may also produce androgens and so cause virilism with associated hirsutism and increasing libido.

18.10 Diabetes insipidus is associated with:

1. the oversecretion of vasopressin
2. polydipsia

3. a urine specific gravity greater than 1020
4. head injury
5. metastatic cancer

1. False
The cause of diabetes insipidus is a deficiency of vasopressin. This causes the uncontrollable diuresis which leads to the accompanying polyuria. Vasopressin alters the responsiveness of the plasma membrane on the luminal surface of the tubular cells.

2. True
The polyuria of diabetes insipidus is accompanied by polydipsia. Increasing thirst leads to a grossly increased intake of water.

3. False
The urine specific gravity in diabetes insipidus rarely rises above 1005.

4. True
A head injury which results in damage to the hypothalamus may result in diabetes insipidus. However, neither destruction of the neurohypophysis nor high transection of the pituitary stalk usually cause diabetes insipidus because sufficient ADH escapes from the severed neurohypophyseal tract.

5. True
If metastatic cancer involves the hypothalamus diabetes insipidus may follow.

Section 19. THE RENAL SYSTEM

19.1 Renal function is depressed in the following conditions:

1. 'Shock'
2. Amyloidosis
3. Chronic hyperuricaemia
4. Irradiation
5. Hypercalcaemia

1. True
'Shock' particularly when due to loss of water and salt or haemorrhage depresses renal function by causing severe renal vasoconstriction. Following

severe blood loss, if the blood volume remains reduced for several hours, the renal vasoconstriction may be sufficiently severe to cause tubular or glomerular necrosis. Fortunately the former is more common and is reversible.

2. True
Amyloidosis, which follows chronic sepsis or rheumatoid arthritis, may also occur as a familial condition. When the kidney is affected proteinuria follows and the nephrotic syndrome develops. Occasionally renal vein thrombosis occurs to produce acute renal failure.

3. True
Chronic hyperuricaemia causes chronic renal failure by the production of interstitial nephritis, nephrosclerosis and possibly the development of uric acid stones.

4. True
If the kidneys are not protected from irradiation, for example, during the treatment of para-aortic glands, they will be damaged. The onset of symptoms often follows a latent interval of six to twelve months after which oedema, dyspnoea, hypertension, headache, nausea and vomiting, lassitude and nocturia occur. Death usually occurs due to hypertensive cardiac failure, hypertensive fits and renal failure.

5. True
Hypercalcaemia leads to hypercalciuria which in turn leads to nephrocalcinosis. At this stage renal function is depressed due to the tubular defect which is produced.

19.2 The renal control of acid base balance is a function of the:

1. loop of Henle
2. proximal tubule
3. glomerulus
4. distal tubule
5. collecting tubule

1. False
2. False

3. False
4. True
5. False

Acids in the body are taken up by buffer system:

$$H^+A + NaHCO_3 \rightleftharpoons Na\ A + H_2CO_3 \rightleftharpoons H_2O + CO_2$$
(acid produced by some
metabolic process)

The carbon dioxide is excreted by the lungs and the anion by the kidney but if this was excreted together with the sodium ion, the net result of the production of one hydrogen ion would be the loss from the body of one molecule of sodium bicarbonate. This depletion is prevented by the formation of carbonic acid within the cells of the distal tubules under the control of carbonic anhydrase. The cell then exchanges hydrogen for sodium in the tubular lumen and sodium bicarbonate is returned to the blood. A further mechanism involved is the production of ammonia by the cells of the distal tubule. The ammonia ion combines with a hydrogen ion and a chloride ion in the tubular lumen, sodium is reabsorbed in exchange and ammonium chloride is excreted in the urine.

19.3 In renal tubular acidosis the following biochemical abnormalities occur:

1. An inability to lower the urine pH
2. Abnormal ammonia excretion in relation to urine pH
3. Renal glycosuria
4. Hypercalciuria
5. Hyperkalaemia

1. True
The inability to lower urine pH is due to an inability to produce and maintain a hydrogen ion gradient between the tubule lumen and the cell. With normal quantities of buffer in the urine the impaired ability to lower the urine pH results in a reduced excretion of titratable acid.

2. False
Ammonia excretion is usually normal in relation to the urine pH, but as the urine pH cannot be reduced

310

the absolute excretion of ammonia is nearly always low.

3. False
Renal glycosuria does not occur.

4. True
Hypercalciuria can occur and may be associated with nephrocalcinosis although they may occur independently. The hypercalciuria is due to the systemic acidosis because the hydrogen ions tend to be buffered by bone with the release of calcium into the extracellular fluid.

5. False
Increased potassium excretion occurs leading to hypokalaemia. This is due to systemic acidosis and also secondary aldosteronism which develops when the affected patients become sodium depleted.

19.4 The nephrotic syndrome is accompanied by:

1. decreased glomerular capillary permeability
2. oedema
3. a loss of 10 g or more of plasma protein daily
4. hypolipidaemia
5. abundant cortical deposits of neutral fat and anisotropic lipids

1. False
The major defect in the nephrotic syndrome is an increase in glomerular capillary permeability. This may occur in various types of glomerulonephritis, e.g. membranoproliferative glomerulonephritis which most commonly occurs in older children.

2. True
Generalised oedema occurs because of the loss of albumin. It should be remembered that conditions other than renal disease may produce the same effect, e.g. protein losing enteropathy and chronic malnutrition.

3. True
It is this huge loss of albumin which leads to the associated generalised oedema by reducing the osmotic pressure in the capillaries.

4. False

For reasons not understood the nephrotic syndrome is associated with hyperlipidaemia. Whereas in a normal individual the normal daily urinary excretion of fats is less than 10 mg in the nephrotic syndrome this may rise to 1000 mg due to the hyperlipidaemia. The crystallisation of cholesterol esters gives rise to the classical birefringent urinary crystals.

5. True

The kidneys in the nephrotic syndrome are enlarged and pallid due to oedema and frequently a yellow, radial streaking of the cortex is present due to the deposition of lipids. Both anisotropic lipid and some sudanophil neutral fat (dark) is deposited in the interstitial tissue and tubules.

19.5 The causes of acute tubular necrosis of the kidney include:

1. severe dehydration
2. the overadministration of carbon tetrachloride
3. acute porphyria
4. the overadministration of potassium chloride
5. gentamicin

1. True

Tubular necrosis follows severe dehydration because of the severe reduction in blood volume which results in renal ischaemia from two causes, first the reduced flow of blood through the kidney and secondly, the accompanying vasoconstriction.

2. True

Carbon tetrachloride is a poison which acts directly on the tubular cells, in addition along with many other poisons it causes intense renal vasoconstriction which results in a patchy tubular necrosis.

3. True

Acute porphyria is often provoked by the administration of barbiturates. At autopsy large amounts of porphyrins can be identified in the tubule cells leading to tubular malfunction.

4. False

The potassium salt which causes renal damage is potassium chlorate. Potassium chloride administration is associated with mucosal ulceration of the small bowel leading to ulceration, possible perforation or stricture formation.

5. False
Gentamicin is not *per se* a cause of renal damage but in the presence of renal damage the continuous administration of this drug is dangerous because of its ototoxic effect. Profound vestibular disturbance occurs.

19.6 The differences between the tubular lesions produced by nephrotoxic drugs and renal ischaemia include:

1. The lesion produced by ischaemia occurs in a random fashion throughout all nephrons and in any part of the nephron down to collecting tubules
2. A nephrotoxic drug affects the entire nephron
3. Nephrotoxic drugs produce scattered lesions throughout the kidney
4. Ischaemia causes complete necrosis of the tubule cell together with the basement membrane
5. Nephrotoxins cause both cytotoxic and ischaemic lesions

1. True
Ischaemic lesions of the kidney are associated with random lesions in which any part of the nephron may be affected.

2. False
Nephrotoxic drugs affect all nephrons equally and the lesions are confined to the same part of each proximal tubule.

3. False
The effect of nephrotoxic drugs is to produce a generalised lesion throughout the kidney.

4. True
Complete necrosis of the tubule cells and the basement membrane exposes the lumen of the tubule to the renal interstitial space.

5. True
Nephrotoxins cause ischaemic lesions because the

cytotoxic agents in high concentration cause intense renal vasoconstriction.

19.7 Uretero-colic anastomosis is followed by:

1. ascending pyelonephritis
2. absorption of ammonium salts
3. absorption of urea from the colon
4. metabolic alkalosis
5. hyperkalaemia

1. True
This operation is invariably followed by the reflux of faecal material up the ureters, causing severe renal infection.

2. True
Ammonium salts are absorbed in excess from the bowel because of the ammonia formed from the urine by the urea splitting bacteria in the colon.

3. True
The reabsorption of urea from the urine by the colon is sufficient, even in the absence of any change in renal function, to cause a rise in the blood urea. It can be distinguished from a rise in blood urea due to a true depression of glomerular filtration by estimating the plasma creatinine since the latter is not absorbed from the bowel.

4. False
Uretero-colic anastomosis is followed by the reabsorption of chloride to a greater extent than sodium ions. This, together with the reabsorption of hydrogen ions, tends to cause an acidosis strictly known as hyperchloraemic acidosis.

5. False
Following ureterocolic anastomosis an excessive loss of potassium occurs probably due to two causes:
   (a) Increased quantities of urinary potassium are delivered into the colon once pyelonephritis develops.
   (b) Excessive loss from the colon itself due to the large amount of colonic mucus which is excreted due to irritation of the wall of the bowel by urine.

19.8 Haemoglobinuria occurs:

1. in blackwater fever
2. following the excessive ingestion of beetroot
3. in any cause of haematuria when the specific gravity of the urine is above 1007
4. in blood transfusion
5. in strenuous exercise

1. True
Blackwater fever is the name given to a complication of malignant tertian malaria. It usually occurs in patients who have been previously treated with antimalarial drugs, particularly quinine, either prophylactically or for recurrent attacks of malaria. Sudden and severe haemolysis occurs followed in some cases by acute renal failure.

2. False
The urine may become red following the eating of beetroot due to the excretion of the red dye vegetable origin.

3. False
Haematuria, the passage of red cells, in the urine has many causes. In the presence of a hypotonic urine when the specific gravity is below 1007 the red cells in the bladder are haemolysed and haemoglobinuria occurs.

4. False
Blood transfusion is not followed by haemoglobinuria unless the transfused blood belongs to the incorrect group. Such mismatched blood is immediately haemolysed, the plasma concentration of haemoglobin rises and there is fever, shivering, severe pains in the back, hypotension and haemoglobinuria.

5. True
Any normal person who undergoes sufficiently severe and prolonged strenuous exercise will develop haemoglobinuria and proteinuria. This has been shown in marathon runners. It is a benign condition and associated with no late sequelae.

Section 20. WATER AND ELECTROLYTE DISTURBANCE

20.1 The major differences between the plasma and the interstitial fluid are in:

315

1. the concentration of sodium
2. the concentration of calcium
3. the bicarbonate concentration
4. the protein content
5. the organic acid concentration

1. True
The concentration of sodium in the former is 152 mmol/l (mEq/l) and in the latter 143 mmol/l (mEq/l).

2. False
The concentration of calcium is the same in both.

3. False
The concentration of bicarbonate ion is the same and equal in both.

4. True
The protein content of the plasma is approximately eight times greater than in the interstitial fluid.

5. False
The concentration of organic acid is the same in both.

20.2 The percentage of total body water in any individual is influenced by:

1. the lean body mass
2. the activity of the adrenal cortex
3. an increased sodium content of the diet
4. thyroid activity
5. vomiting

1. True
The total body water in a normal individual is particularly related to lean body mass. Since the lean body mass is greater in the male but decreases with age in both sexes the percentage of body water is always greater in the male than the female at any age.

2. True
Cortical hyperplasia or benign or malignant cortical tumours leading to the secretion of abnormal quantities of cortisol cause the retention of sodium and water.

3. False
Excessive quantities of sodium in the diet are absorbed and then excreted by the kidney due to diminished tubular reabsorption.

4. True
Overactivity of the thyroid, i.e. thyrotoxicosis, leads to proximal muscle wasting and hence loss of lean body mass. Indirectly, therefore, thyrotoxicosis must be associated with a reduction in the percentage of total body water. Underactivity of the thyroid, however, which is associated with myxoedema, is associated with an increase in the mucopolysaccharides of the ground substance.

5. True
Persistent vomiting causes a reduction in extracellular fluid and hence of the percentage of total body water.

20.3 The renin-angiotensin-aldosterone system regulates:

1. potassium balance
2. sodium balance
3. fluid volume
4. blood pressure
5. nitrogen balance

1. True
Aldosterone acts to promote K^+ loss at the same time stimulating Na^+ reabsorption by the Na^+–K^+ ion exchange transport system. As the plasma potassium falls, aldosterone secretion is accordingly reduced.

2. True
Because sodium depletion is followed by a contraction of the effective blood volume and a fall in the arterial pressure renal perfusion diminishes and as a result renin is secreted into the blood stream. Renin then acts enzymatically on a plasma globulin causing the release of angiotensin I which is rapidly hydrolysed to angiotensin II. The latter in addition to its pressor action stimulates aldosterone secretion which then acts on the distal tubules to produce sodium retention.

317

3. True

The positive sodium balance induced by adrenal cortical aldosterone secretion increases the volume of extracellular water and in addition enhances the pressor activity of angiotensin.

4. True

Renin, by way of angiotensin, has a pressor effect which is mediated mainly by peripheral vasoconstriction.

5. False

This system has no direct effect on nitrogen balance.

20.4 The blood urea is elevated in the following conditions:

1. Severe dehydration
2. Pregnancy
3. Tubular necrosis
4. Diabetes insipidus
5. Cortical necrosis

1. True

Severe dehydration eventually leads to a fall in the effective blood volume which is followed by hypotension and a diminution in the renal perfusion. At first a physiological diminution in the urine output occurs which can be corrected if the underlying dehydration is rapidly and effectively dealt with. If, however, the condition is not corrected tubular or cortical necrosis follows.

2. False

In pregnancy a low blood urea is commonplace because of the relative increase in blood volume.

3. True

Tubular necrosis is followed by severe oliguria and the retention of urea. Rarely the volume of urine may be as great or greater than normal but urea retention still occurs. This condition is known as non-oliguric renal failure and is particularly seen following severe burns.

4. False

Diabetes insipidus, caused by damage to the hypothalamus or the posterior portion of the hypophysis, is normally not associated with changes in the blood urea.

5. True
Cortical necrosis is followed by an immediate rise in blood urea and complete anuria. The condition is irreversible and requires intermittent dialysis or renal transplantation to maintain life.

20.5 Combined water and electrolyte depletion causes:

1. a high concentration of sodium in the urine
2. a high urine specific gravity
3. pre-renal uraemia
4. a fall in the central venous pressure
5. a high blood urea nitrogen to creatinine ratio

1. False
A combined water and electrolyte depletion results in an augmented secretion of aldosterone which causes an increase in the tubular reabsorption of sodium and hence a low urinary sodium concentration.

2. True
The conservation of water by the kidney results in the excretion of a hypertonic urine. The specific gravity rises above 1020 and the osmolality exceeds 500 mOsm/l.

3. True
The diminishing blood volume results in a gradual decline in renal perfusion and hence a diminished excretion of urea. The retention of urea eventually leads to pre-renal uraemia.

4. True
The decrease in blood volume eventually leads to a decline in the central venous pressure following the exhaustion of the compensatory mechanisms.

5. False
The pre-renal uraemia associated with water and electrolyte depletion causes a disproportionate rise in the blood urea nitrogen as compared to the rising concentration of creatinine. The normal ratio be-

tween these substances is 10:1 but in severe depletion may rise to levels as high as 20 or 25:1.

20.6 Pure water depletion in the surgical patient follows:

1. persistent vomiting
2. dysphagia
3. severe diarrhoea
4. persistent fever
5. the development of diabetes insipidus

1. False
Persistent vomiting results in a combined water and
electrolyte depletion because of the electrolytes
present in the gastrointestinal juices. Gastric juice,
for example, contains between 70 and 140 mEq/l
(mmol/l) of sodium and between 5 and 40 mEq/l
(mmol/l) of potassium.

2. True
Dysphagia caused, for example, by benign or malignant strictures of the oesophagus results, if sufficiently severe, in the regurgitation of all water taken
by mouth in addition to the loss of saliva. The result
is a pure water depletion because fluid rather than
electrolytes is lost.

3. False
Severe diarrhoea gives rise to a combined depletion
in which the loss of potassium is of great importance
because diarrhoeal stools contain between 10 and 40
mEq/l (10 to 40 mmol/l) of this cation. The loss of
approximately 10 per cent of the total body potassium causes the serum potassium to fall from 4 mEq/l
(mmol/l) to 3 mEq/l (mmol/l) at a normal pH.

4. True
Fever is associated with increased sweating. This is
the major mechanism of heat loss but is only effective
if the sweat evaporates on the skin surface, thus
extracting the latent heat of vaporisation. Excessive
sweating causes a pure water depletion but if the
water is replaced alone salt deficiency follows.

5. True
Diabetes insipidus follows a reduction, from whatever cause, of circulating vasopressin. A vasopressin

deficiency results in the excretion of large volumes of dilute urine due to an alteration in the response of the tubular cells to the movement of water. Between 5 and 10 litres/day of urine may be excreted daily leading rapidly, unless corrected, by a corresponding increase in water intake, to water depletion.

20.7 The metabolic effects following a severe injury include:

1. respiratory alkalosis
2. accelerated gluconeogenesis
3. mobilisation of fat stores
4. decreased aldosterone secretion
5. protein anabolism

1. True
Respiratory alkalosis may follow the hyperventilation induced by pain and blood loss.

2. True
Afferent stimuli reaching the central nervous system through large neurones causes the hypothalamus to secrete corticotrophin releasing factor (CRF). The resulting stimulation of the anterior pituitary releases adrenotrophic hormone (ACTH). This, in turn, stimulates the excessive secretion of glucocorticoids by the adrenal cortex which accelerates gluconeogenesis and increases the deposition of liver glycogen.

3. True
The mobilisation of fat stores from adipose tissue elevates the serum levels of free fatty acids. The net effect is to increase the plasma concentration of carbohydrate and lipid intermediates producing the 'diabetes of injury'.

4. False
Aldosterone secretion may be increased almost thirty-fold following severe trauma. This enhances the renal tubular absorption of sodium thus helping to maintain the extracellular fluid volume. In addition the excretion of hydrogen ion and potassium are increased thus delaying the onset of a metabolic acidosis and hyperkalaemia.

5. False
Trauma from whatever cause induces protein catabolism. Normally an individual receiving no protein
in the diet excretes nitrogen at an accelerated rate of
10 to 12 g/day for about 14 days after which a gradual
decline occurs. In contrast, following major trauma
and in the same dietary conditions the excretion of
nitrogen may reach 20 g/day and if in addition there
is superadded sepsis the nitrogen excretion may
reach 30 g/day. This is equivalent to the loss of 180 g
of protein daily or 1 kg (wet weight) of body tissue.

20.8 Hyperkalaemia commonly occurs:

1. following severe burns
2. in Conn's syndrome
3. following glomerular necrosis
4. in the Zollinger–Ellison syndrome
5. in the carcinoid syndrome

1. True
Hyperkalaemia occurs in severe burns due to the
following factors:
  (a) Liberation of potassium from the haemolysis
      of the erythrocytes destroyed or damaged in
      the burnt area
  (b) Associated tissue catabolism
  (c) Retention of potassium due to renal failure

2. False
This uncommon syndrome, which is usually caused
by aldosterone secreting tumours of the adrenal
cortex, is associated with the retention of sodium
and the excessive excretion of potassium leading to
hypokalaemia.

3. True
Glomerular necrosis, however caused, results in irreversible renal failure and the retention of potassium.

4. False
The Zollinger–Ellison syndrome caused by gastrin
secreting tumours of the islet cells of the pancreas
may be associated with severe diarrhoea. Should this
occur water and electrolyte depletion follows and

hyperkalaemia would only occur if secondary renal failure developed.

5. False
The carcinoid syndrome may be associated with diarrhoea but this is normally episodic and rarely sufficiently severe to produce electrolyte depletion.

20.9 Hypocalcaemia occurs:

1. following surgical damage or removal of the parathyroid glands
2. following fractures of the long bones
3. during attacks of acute pancreatitis
4. following head injury
5. in association with hypomagnesaemia

1. True
Hypocalcaemia follows damage to the parathyroid glands during the operation of thyroidectomy. Some surgeons argue that the cause is removal of the glands, others that it is due to damage to their arterial supply leading to infarction. Whatever the precise cause the end result is a diminished supply of parathyroid hormone and tetany follows.

2. False
Simple fractures of the long bones do not affect the serum calcium.

3. True
Severe pancreatitis is associated with the liberation of the enzyme, lipase. This specifically hydrolyses fat, especially within the abdomen, the liberated soaps combine with calcium causing acute hypocalcaemia. If this does occur in pancreatitis it is regarded as a bad prognostic sign.

4. False
Although severe trauma may be associated with hypocalcaemia head injury alone does not produce this metabolic disturbance.

5. True
Hypomagnesaemia is frequently associated with hypocalcaemia. This is due to the fact that both electrolyte disturbances may share a common aetiology, i.e. malabsorption from whatever cause.

20.10 Severe pyloric stenosis is accompanied by the following biochemical changes:

1. A fall in the effective blood volume
2. A fall in the concentration of plasma sodium
3. A rise in pCO_2
4. Hypotonic urine
5. Hyperkalaemia

1. True
The continuous loss of water accompanied by sodium and chloride reduces the volume of all fluid spaces including the blood volume. The net result on the kidney is renal vasoconstriction and a reduced glomerular filtration rate, as a result the blood urea is elevated.

2. False
Although there is an overall sodium deficiency due to vomiting the vomitus contains relatively more water than sodium so that the concentration of plasma sodium sometimes rises. If, however, the patient is allowed to drink, the selective partial replacement of water to the exclusion of sodium lowers the plasma concentration of sodium below normal.

3. True
The loss of hydrogen ions raises the plasma pH, slows respiration and raises the pCO_2.

4. False
The normal change in the urine is oliguria associated with a hypertonic urine. If renal ischaemia is severe tubular necrosis follows.

5. False
The continuous vomiting leads to a low plasma potassium and to compensate for this a potassium shift occurs from the intracellular space to the plasma and extracellular space, together with a reverse shift of hydrogen and sodium ions from the extracellular space into the cells.

Section 21. BLOOD TRANSFUSION

21.1 Blood which is to be used for transfusion:

1. should be stored at −4°C

2. may need to be irradiated (1000 r)
3. needs to be tested for complement content
4. may be used after storage for platelet replacement
5. should be stored in an acid anticoagulant

1. False
Blood transfusion should be stored at +4°C. If frozen the erythrocytes will be lysed releasing haemoglobin into the plasma. The introduction of lysed blood into a recipient can give rise to an immediate transfusion reaction accompanied by haemoglobinaemia, haemoglobinuria and possibly oliguria followed by acute renal failure.

2. True
Fresh blood transfused to an immunodeficient patient should be irradiated to prevent a graft versus host reaction.

3. False
Stored blood does not contain very much active complement and is not normally checked for circulating immune complexes.

4. False
If platelet replacement is required fresh blood must be used as platelets decay rapidly. Platelet transfusions are required in cases of bone marrow aplasia and acute leukaemia. If, however, platelet autoantibodies have developed or if increased destruction of platelets is occurring in the spleen, platelet transfusion will be ineffective.

5. True
The standard anticoagulant used for donor blood is acid citrate dextrose. This is a mixture of citric acid, trisodium citrate and dextrose, acidification increasing the preserving power of the solution.

21.2 The following tests should be performed on donor blood before it is used for transfusion:

1. HbsAg
2. Van den Bergh
3. Wassermann test or the VDRL flocculation test
4. Acid phosphatase
5. Malaria smear

1. True

The presence of HBsAg (Australia antigen) in donor blood means that there is a high risk of transferring hepatitis B infection to the recipient. This antigen may be identified by a variety of methods including gel precipitation and counterimmuno-electrophoresis.

2. False

The Van den Bergh diazo test for bilirubin is not routinely performed on donor blood prior to transfusion.

3. True

In the presence of a positive Wassermann or VDRL flocculation reaction there is a risk of the transfused blood transferring syphilis. Thus Wassermann or VDRL positive blood should not be used for transfusion.

4. False

The acid phosphatase in serum is raised in prostatic cancer with osteoplastic secondary deposits in bone.

5. True

In tropical countries in which malaria is endemic there is always a risk of transfusing blood containing malaria parasites; a smear should, therefore, be examined to exclude this disease in donor blood.

21.3 The following refer to blood group antigens:

1. Lewis
2. Von Willebrand
3. Duffy
4. Turner
5. Kidd

1. True

Lewis antigens Le^a and Le^b are associated with the red cells and are also found in the saliva and plasma. The system is controlled by the genes Le and le. There is a connection between the Lewis system and the ability to secrete blood group substances. Lewis antibodies are not associated with haemolytic disease of the newborn since they belong to the IgM group and, therefore, cannot cross the placenta.

2. False
Von Willebrand's disease is a hereditary clotting disorder similar to haemophilia. The deficiency is in clotting Factor VIII but, in addition, an increased bleeding time occurs due to capillary fragility. Clinically, the condition presents with mucosal bleeding as well as repeated attacks of haemarthrosis.

3. True
The Duffy system (Fy^a positive and Fy^a negative) give rise to IgG antibodies that can pass across the placenta and give rise to haemolytic disease of the newborn. Anti-Fy^a antibodies are best detected by a Coombs test.

4. False
Turner's syndrome is due to the absence of the Y chromosome and a single X chromosome. It is associated with ovarian dysgenesis, a lack of sexual development and a webbed neck.

5. True
The Kidd system (Jk^a positive and Jk^a negative) is similar to the Duffy and Kell blood group systems. These antigens can also result in IgG antibodies causing severe haemolytic disease of the newborn.

21.4 An immediate reaction to a blood transfusion may be caused by the following:

1. Hypercalcaemia
2. Air embolus
3. Bacterial endotoxins
4. Anaphylaxis
5. Hypokalaemia

1. False
A transfusion of blood does not give rise to hypercalcaemia. However, the transfusion of large volumes of stored blood may give rise to hypocalcaemia due to the action of the citrate which is used as an anticoagulant. This effect can be reversed by the administration of calcium gluconate.

2. True
Air embolus is a recognised risk of any transfusion administered by a donor set with interchangeable

parts. Much of this risk has been removed by the use of plastic packs.

3. True
Fever was a common complication of blood transfusion in the past. It arose either because the blood had been contaminated by bacterial endotoxins or because residual pyrogens had been absorbed onto the donor apparatus. Many of these latter reactions have been eliminated by the use of plastic disposable donor sets.

4. True
Anaphylactic reaction following transfusion gives rise to urticaria. The responsible antigens are probably derived from food ingested immediately prior to taking the blood, examples being bovine milk and egg proteins.

5. False
Massive transfusions lead to hyperkalaemia; this can cause heart failure and possibly sudden death.

21.5 The physical results of rhesus incompatibility include the following:

1. Hydrops foetalis
2. Hutchinson's teeth
3. Icterus neonatorum
4. Hepato-lenticular degeneration
5. Kernicterus

1. True
Severe rhesus incompatibility results in hydrops foetalis, a cause of intrauterine death due to the development of marked anaemia and congestive heart failure, the latter causing severe oedema, hence the name.

2. False
Hutchinson's teeth have no connection with rhesus incompatibility, they are one of the many stigmata of congenital syphilis.

3. True
Extreme incompatibility causes such a severe degree of intravascular haemolysis that the affected baby is deeply jaundiced at birth.

4. False

Hepato-lenticular degeneration, Wilson's disease, has no connection with rhesus incompatibility. It is a familial disease of children caused by an excess of free copper in the circulation due to the low levels of the copper binding caeruloplasmin in the circulation. Copper is deposited in the brain particularly in the putamen and caudate nucleus and also in the liver and kidneys.

5. True

The severe haemolysis which may occur in rhesus incompatibility results in jaundice causing the condition known as kernicterus in which staining of the hippocampus and basal nuclei with bile occurs. This leads to localised brain damage with necrosis of the affected neurones which is later followed by gliosis. If not fatal the child is likely to suffer from choreo-athetosis, spasticity and mental deficiency.

21.6 Haemolytic disease of the newborn:

1. may be caused by *Treponema pallidum*
2. may be due to anti-c
3. may occur in the first pregnancy
4. frequently is not found until the second pregnancy
5. is treated with anti-D antibodies

1. False

Treponema pallidum plays no part in haemolytic disease of the newborn which is chiefly caused by rhesus incompatibility and rarely to ABO incompatibility.

2. True

Rhesus incompatibility is usually due to anti-D but rarely it can be due to either anti-c or anti-E.

3. True

HDN can occur in the first pregnancy but only if the mother has previously received an Rh incompatible transfusion.

4. True

The first pregnancy is usually uneventful, the Rh negative mother being delivered at term of an Rh positive child without any apparent difficulties.

However, the first pregnancy leads to immunisation of the mother so that when a second pregnancy occurs the anti Rh maternal antibodies reach the fetus via the placental circulation and varying degrees of HDN occur.

5. True
This condition can be prevented by the administration of 200 to 300 μg anti Rh antibody by intramuscular injection to the mother. The passively injected antibody probably acts as a negative feedback turning off antibody production.

21.7 The Coombs test is used for detecting:

1. rheumatoid factor
2. antinuclear factor
3. haemolytic autoantibodies
4. cold agglutinins
5. rhesus antibodies

1. False
The Coombs test uses an antihuman globulin antibody to detect specific immunoglobulins or complement attached to, or capable of attaching to, the surface of human erythrocytes. The rheumatoid factor is, however, an antibody directed towards the Gm groups on the Fc fragment of immunoglobulins. It is detected either by using sensitised sheep erythrocytes (Rose–Waaler test) or latex particles onto which human IgG has been absorbed.

2. False
The antinuclear factor is an autoantibody chiefly present in the serum of patients suffering from systemic lupus erythematosus. It is detected either by a latex test in which the antigen is absorbed onto latex particles or by immunofluorescent techniques.

3. True
The direct Coombs test detects antibodies that have already reacted with antigen on the red cell surface. The indirect Coombs test is used to detect antibodies to red cell antigens present in serum which are first reacted with specific red cells before the application of antihuman globulin reagent. The test produces red cell agglutination.

4. True

The Coombs test will detect agglutinins that have reacted with the surface of the erythrocyte even if the reaction occurs at 37°C.

5. True

The presence of IgG (incomplete) rhesus antibodies in the serum can be detected by the use of an indirect Coombs test.

21.8 The following antibodies may pass across the placenta:

1. Anti A isohaemagglutinin
2. Immune antiblood group A
3. Anti D (rhesus)
4. Diphtheria antitoxin
5. Rheumatoid factor

1. False

The anti ABO blood group antibodies present in normal plasma are IgM antibodies (MW 900 000) too large to pass across the placenta.

2. True

The immune anti ABO blood group antibodies which may develop after a transfusion of incompatible blood are sometimes of IgG type and may, therefore, pass across the placenta to cause haemolytic disease of the newborn.

3. True

Anti D (rhesus) antibodies formed following rhesus positive pregnancies in rhesus negative mothers or an incompatible transfusion in a rhesus negative mother are usually of IgG type and, therefore, pass across the placenta.

4. True

Diphtheria antitoxin is an IgG antibody which, therefore, passes across the placenta.

5. False

The rheumatoid factor is an IgM anti IgG autoantibody developing in individuals suffering from rheumatoid arthritis and does not pass across the placenta.

Section 22. IONISING IRRADIATION AND CYTOTOXIC AGENTS

22.1 Ionising radiation:

1. increases DNA synthesis
2. increases H_2O_2 in the tissues
3. breaks disulphide bonds
4. causes atrophy of the seminiferous tubules of the testis
5. causes pathological fractures

1. False
X-irradiation causes a decrease in DNA synthesis, which results in a diminution in the rate of mitoses and a slowing down of cell turnover.

2. True
Oxidising compounds such as H_2O_2 are formed. This gives rise to oxidation of -SH groups to -S-S- groups.

3. False
Disulphide bonds are formed rather than broken following irradiation. This causes the inactivation of enzymes which contain -SH groups as part of their biochemically active sites.

4. True
The first effect of irradiation on the testes is the destruction of the spermatogonia. A later effect is atrophy of the seminiferous tubules.

5. True
Bone is affected in two ways by irradiation, firstly radionecrosis may occur and secondly, late ischaemia may be followed by fractures particularly of the pelvis and femur.

22.2 The effect(s) of ionising irradiation:

1. are increased by sulphydryl reagents
2. are increased by increased oxygen tension
3. is mainly upon mitochondria
4. is to cause diarrhoea
5. is to cause a deficiency of clotting factors

1. False
See answer to question 2.

2. True

An increase in the oxygen tension in the environment of a malignant tumour increases the tumoricidal effects of irradiation. Much of this effect is believed to be caused by the oxidation of the -SH groups of enzymes to -S-S- groups, thus inactivating enzyme activity. In animal tumour systems sulphydryl containing compounds such as cysteine, cysteamine and AET afford some protection from the effects of irradiation.

3. False

There is no doubt that irradiation has an effect on the mitochondrial enzymes but its major effect is to inhibit DNA synthesis and mitosis, thus the main effect of ionising irradiation on any cell is at a nuclear level.

4. True

Irradiation of the abdominal cavity will lead to necrosis of the gastro-intestinal mucosa if the dose is sufficiently high, i.e. above 800 r. If this occurs a bloody diarrhoea follows which may be sufficiently severe to cause dehydration and shock.

5. False

Ionising irradiation may be followed by severe bleeding but if this occurs it is due to a platelet deficiency caused by a direct radiation effect on the megakaryocytes of the bone marrow. A bleeding tendency may develop within about two weeks of irradiation following doses in the region of 450 r.

22.3 Ionising radiation:

1. does not affect the eyes
2. affects renal function
3. does not affect the lungs
4. affects the brain
5. does not affect the skin

1. False

Large doses of irradiation, particularly by neutrons, can cause cataracts.

2. True

Excessive exposure of the kidneys to ionising irradiation causes a progressive glomerular fibrosis which leads to malignant hypertension and a progressive diminution of renal function.

3. False
Ionising irradiation does affect the lungs causing pulmonary fibrosis and a decline in respiratory function. This was a relatively common complication following the treatment of carcinoma of the breast prior to the use of high energy irradiation and tangential fields.

4. True
Very high doses in excess of 5000 r may be associated with a cerebral syndrome in which hyperthermia followed by a state of shock occurs.

5. False
Ionising irradiation gives rise to an inflammatory response which is later followed by atrophy of the skin and hypopigmentation and subsequently the development of squamous carcinomata, and/or rodent ulcers.

22.4 The following are immunosuppressive drugs:

1. Azathioprine
2. Indomethacin
3. Oxyprenolol
4. Cyclophosphamide
5. Chlorpropamide

1. True
Azathioprine, a guanine analogue based on 6-mercaptopurine, is the most widely used immunosuppressive drug in clinical practice. It is part of the standard drug regime used to prevent graft rejection in renal transplantation patients and it is also occasionally used in the treatment of autoimmune diseases such as systemic lupus erythematosus.

2. False
Indomethacin is an anti-inflammatory drug without any direct immunosuppressive action. It is chiefly used in the treatment of rheumatoid arthritis. Indomethacin inhibits the formation of prostaglandins from the substrate arachidonic acid.

3. False
Oxyprenolol and propanolol are β adrenergic recep-

tor blockers and are used in the treatment of cardiac arrhythmias and hypertension.

4. True

Cyclophosphamide is an alkylating agent derived from nitrogen mustard. As a cytotoxic drug it is chiefly used in the treatment of neoplastic disease but it is cytotoxic to all rapidly dividing cells and, therefore, to the lymphocytes concerned in the immune response, although it is not particularly effective in preventing graft rejection.

5. False

Chlorpropamide is an oral antidiabetic agent. It reduces the blood sugar by increasing the cellular uptake of glucose and decreasing the intestinal absorption of sugars.

22.5 The following compounds may be used as anti-cancer agents:

1. Azathioprine
2. Methotrexate
3. Actinomycin D
4. Chlorambucil
5. Cyclosporin A

1. False

Azathioprine (Imuran) is an immunosuppressive agent which is commonly used to suppress transplant rejection and occasionally for the treatment of autoimmune immune complex diseases, such as systemic lupus erythematosus. It is not an anticancer agent.

2. True

Methotrexate is a folic acid inhibitor used in the treatment of leukaemia. It has also been used as an immunosuppressive agent and also to suppress the epidermal proliferation which occurs in psoriasis.

3. True

The actinomycins are antibiotics which suppress proliferating tissue in man. Actinomycin D selectively complexes with DNA and thus inhibits RNA and protein synthesis. This antibiotic is particularly effective in the treatment of childhood renal tumours. Actinomycin C which contains some actinomycin D has been used in combination with azathioprine to prevent the rejection of renal transplants.

4. True
Aminophenylbutyric acid mustard (chlorambucil) is an alkylating agent which has been used to suppress cellular and particularly neoplastic proliferation.

5. False
Cyclosporin A is a fungal metabolite which acts as an immunosuppressive agent by its action on the T-lymphocytes. It has been used to treat renal allograft recipients and to prevent graft versus host disease after bone marrow transplantation.

22.6 The following compounds are alkylating agents:

1. Azathioprine
2. Methotrexate
3. Cyclophosphamide
4. Phenylalanine mustard
5. Tetracycline

1. False
Azathioprine (Imuran) is the carrier form of 6-mercaptopurine which is incorporated into DNA instead of guanine as a fraudulent base.

2. False
Methotrexate is a folic acid inhibitor blocking DNA synthesis.

3. True
Cyclophosphamide is not strictly an alkylating agent but it is broken down by the liver *in vivo* to liberate nitrogen mustard which is an alkylating agent.

4. True
L phenyl alanine mustard (Melphalan) is an alkylating agent. Great hopes were once entertained that this drug would be successful in the cure of malignant melanoma because it was considered that the phenyl alanine would be incorporated into the melanoma cells as a precursor of melanin. These high hopes were soon dashed.

5. False
Tetracycline is a broad spectrum antibiotic prepared from chlortetracycline, its action is that of a bacteriostatic agent.

22.7 The following immunosuppressive agents are purine or pyrimidine analogues:

1. Cyclophosphamide
2. Azathioprine
3. Methotrexate
4. Actinomycin C
5. Prednisone

1. False
Cyclophosphamide is a derivative of nitrogen mustard. It exerts its cytotoxic effect as an alkylating agent cross linking the DNA double helix.

2. True
Azathioprine which is commonly used following renal transplantation is a derivative of 6 mercaptopurine which is an analogue of the purine base guanine disturbing the DNA sequence which following this cannot be transcribed thus effectively blocking protein synthesis.

3. False
Methotrexate is a folic acid analogue blocking the action of the enzyme folic reductase. As a result, dihydrofolinic acid cannot be reduced to tetrahydrofolinic acid. This is a necessary step for the conversion of uracil desoxyriboside to thymidine, the latter being an essential constituent of DNA.

4. False
Actinomycin C is an antibiotic derived from cultures of *Streptomyces antibioticus*. It selectively competes with DNA inhibiting RNA and protein synthesis. This agent was in the past used to supplement azathioprine in renal transplantation and one of its components actinomycin D is still used for the treatment of renal tumours of childhood.

5. False
Prednisone is a glucocorticoid. The mechanism by which glucocorticoids act as immunosuppressive

agents in man is poorly understood. However, they have a strong anti-inflammatory component.

22.8 Chlorambucil, a potent cytotoxic agent, causes:

1. a cessation of DNA synthesis
2. indirect interference with mitosis
3. inhibition of purine synthesis
4. binding of DNA strands
5. inhibition of protein synthesis

1. False
Synthesis of DNA is inhibited by the antimitotic antibiotics which attach themselves by hydrogen bonds to the guanine moiety of the DNA chain thus preventing DNA synthesis.

2. True
By binding the DNA strands together chlorambucil indirectly interferes with mitosis, see **4**. This action should be compared to the mode of action of the vinca alkaloids which arrest cell division at the metaphase probably by interfering with spindle formation so that the chromatids cannot be properly paired.

3. False
The chief inhibitors of purine synthesis are the nitrosoureas which block the enzymes responsible for purine synthesis and the incorporation of purine into DNA.

4. True
Chlorambucil is an alkylating agent and its cytotoxicity is effected by the development of cross linkages or bridges between opposite guanine bases. This binds the DNA strands together and prevents them from separating at the time of division.

5. True
Inhibition of protein synthesis is an essential feature of the action of all alkylating cytotoxic agents.

22.9 DNA synthesis is inhibited by:

1. prednisone
2. methane sulphonic acid
3. methotrexate

4. azathioprine
5. chloramphenicol

1. False
Glucocorticoids do not directly affect DNA synthesis. They are neither antimitotic agents nor inhibitors of protein synthesis.

2. True
Methane sulphonic acid (Busulphan), is an alkylating agent used in cancer chemotherapy. This agent is believed to form alkyl bridges across the DNA double helix thus inhibiting normal DNA replication.

3. True
Methotrexate is an inhibitor of folic acid which binds the enzyme, folic reductase, thus preventing the reduction of dihydrofolinic acid to tetrahydrofolinic acid. The latter acts as a coenzyme for the conversion of uracil desoxyriboside into thymidine, which is necessary for DNA synthesis.

4. True
Azathioprine (Imuran) is a carrier form of 6 mercaptopurine. It is incorporated into the DNA molecule as a 'fraudulent' base in place of guanine thus preventing the normal synthesis of DNA.

5. False
Chloramphenicol is a broad spectrum antibiotic which was originally obtained from *Streptomyces venezuelae* but is now artificially synthesised. It prevents protein synthesis by mammalian cells by blocking the formation of peptide chains from amino acids on the ribosomes. In addition it may also block the synthesis of messenger RNA in proliferating cells.

Section 23. MISCELLANEOUS

23.1 The following are referred to as 'Incomplete antibodies':

1. IgG anti-D
2. IgM anti-D
3. Anti-A isohaemagglutinin
4. The Wassermann antibody
5. Tetanus antitoxin

1. True
IgG anti-D antibodies will not agglutinate D-positive erythrocytes in a saline solution alone. They require a colloid solution such as 30 per cent bovine albumin or alternatively they can be detected by the use of the indirect Coombs test.

2. False
IgM anti-D antibodies will agglutinate D-positive erythrocytes in saline alone and they are, therefore, referred to as 'complete' antibodies. The terms 'complete' and 'incomplete' are used by haematologists to describe blood group antibodies only. The terms do not mean that structural deficiencies are present in the immunoglobulin molecule. Differences in reaction are probably a function of physical chemical forces.

3. False
Anti-A isohaemagglutinin is an IgM molecule and agglutinates blood group A erythrocytes directly in saline.

4. False
The Wassermann antibody is an IgM antibody which is present in individuals suffering from syphilis and other chronic infectious diseases. It is directed against an antigen present in cholesterolised extracts of bovine heart muscle, and is detected by a complement fixation test.

5. False
Tetanus antitoxin is demonstrated mainly by toxin neutralisation assay in mice. It can also be titrated by passive haemagglutination assay in which tetanus toxoid is bound to a red cell carrier.

23.2 The 'sick cell syndrome' is associated with:

1. cardiac failure prior to surgery or trauma
2. failure of the sodium pump
3. a rise in the urinary sodium excretion
4. apathy
5. intracellular oedema

1. True
The 'sick cell syndrome' is specifically associated with operative intervention or trauma in patients

who have suffered from cardiac failure over a prolonged period.

2. True
The underlying pathology of this syndrome appears
to be a failure of the sodium pump at cell membranes
throughout the body. The result is the passage of
sodium into the intracellular space and the leakage of
potassium.

3. False
Sodium excretion by the kidney diminishes but the
excretion of potassium rises.

4. True
The classic clinical picture of the sick cell syndrome
is one of weakness and apathy developing on the
third or fourth post-operative day. This is accompanied by a fall in the cardiac output, a poor peripheral
circulation, bradycardia and a reduced digoxin tolerance.

5. True
The movement of sodium into the cells causes osmotic swelling to occur associated with the accumulation of water in the cytoplasm and separation of the
organelles.

**23.3 The chief pathological and physiological
changes in 'shock lung' include:**

1. intra-alveolar oedema and extravasation of erythrocytes into the alveoli
2. increased pulmonary compliance
3. infection
4. alkalosis
5. patchy opacities on the plain X-ray of the chest

1. True
Intra-alveolar oedema is the predominant change in
the shock lung syndrome and leads, if sufficiently
severe, to respiratory failure. In addition erythrocyte
extravasation occurs.

2. False
Pulmonary compliance decreases in the 'shock lung'
due to the combination of oedema and extravasation
of erythrocytes. Because of this intermittent positive

pressure ventilation may fail to produce any improvement in the oxygen tension.

3. True
Infection is a common complication of shock lung. Bronchopneumonic change occurs adding an element of toxaemia to the general picture.

4. False
Acidosis accompanies the shock lung and this may be irreversible despite therapy.

5. True
The typical radiological picture of a shock lung is one of patchy opacities. These are attributed to a mixture of pulmonary oedema and collapse.

23.4 The compensatory mechanisms available to preserve the organism as a whole in the 'shock state' include:

1. autoregulation
2. a fall in the pO_2 of the blood
3. decreased pulmonary compliance
4. an increased sympatho-adrenal discharge
5. haemoconcentration

1. True
Autoregulation is the ability of an organ to maintain an adequate blood flow despite changes in the perfusion pressure. It is an intrinsic property of the smooth muscle of the blood vessels of the organ concerned and does not require the intervention of vasomotor nerves. Autoregulation occurs in the cerebral, coronary and renal vascular beds in which steady-state pressure-flow curves are seen until the systolic blood pressure is reduced to approximately 50 mmHg. Below this level a precipitous decline in blood flow follows.

2. False
A fall in the pO_2 does occur in severe shock but this is not a compensatory mechanism. The decrease in oxygen saturation of the systemic blood develops because oxygen has been extracted in such large amounts from the blood returning to the heart from the stagnating circulation. An additional factor in the

later stages is the development of large right to left shunting.

3. False
Decreased compliance of the lungs may occur in severe shock but this is not a compensatory mechanism but a severe disadvantage to the shocked patient leading to the acute respiratory distress syndrome.

4. True
Increased sympatho-adrenal discharge results in increased myocardial contractility and constriction of the arterioles, both factors which tend to restore the blood pressure to normal levels. In addition, the added constriction of the capacitance vessels helps to maintain the venous return to the heart.

5. False
Increased blood viscosity occurs due to loss of the intravascular fluid but this is disadvantageous because it increases the resistance to blood flow particularly in the smaller blood vessels. Eventually widespread aggregation of red cells and platelets occurs, the sludging of blood, a phenomenon first described by Kniseley.

23.5 Which among the following are protozoal infections:

1. Hydatid disease
2. Trypanosomiasis
3. Giardiasis
4. Schistosomiasis
5. Filariasis

1. False
Hydatid disease is caused by a cestode, tapeworm, known as *Echinococcus granulosus* which is transmitted by dogs to man by faecal–oral contamination. The dog is infected by the eating of infected sheep, cattle or pig offal. Man ingests the ova which have a chitinous coat which is digested by the gastric juice thus liberating the embryos. These then invade the veins of the gastrointestinal tract and reach the liver via the portal blood, where most of them lodge to develop into unilocular or multilocular cysts.

2. True

The trypanosomes, *T. gambiense* and *rhodesiense* are both flagellated protozoa. Both are a cause of sleeping sickness, a disease transmitted by the tsetse fly. In South America another species, *T. cruzii*, which is transmitted by the blood sucking bugs of the family *Triatomidae*, causes a condition known as Chagas disease in which severe myocardial damage may occur.

3. True

Giardiasis is caused by the flagellate protozoa *Giardia lamblia*. This parasite causes an intestinal infection which leads to chronic diarrhoea and possible malabsorption.

4. False

Schistosomiasis is caused by a group of trematode worms which infect man after they have been released from their intermediate host. *Schistosoma haematobium* has as its intermediate host the snail, *Bulinus*, which lives in fresh but stagnant water. From the snail free swimming cercariae emerge which enter the human host chiefly through the skin of the legs and also through the mucous membrane of the mouth and pharynx. The adult worms finally reach the vesicle plexus of veins where they settle and pair. The major causes of damage are the ova which are produced. A granulomatous reaction is provoked with the result that fibrosis of bladder wall occurs. In addition squamous metaplasia of the urothelium may be followed by a squamous carcinoma. Another variety, the *Schistosoma mansoni*, inhabit the venules of the lower gastrointestinal tract provoking a granulomatous reaction with subsequent ulceration and melaena. Both may cause pipe-stem periportal fibrosis of the liver which may finally terminate in the development of portal hypertension and oesophageal varices.

5. False

Filariasis is a nematode infection, four different species of filaria can be found in human tissues. The diagnosis of filariasis is made by demonstrating the presence of microfilariae in blood films at night in the case of *Wuchereria bancrofti* or in skin snip biopsies in the case of *Onchocerca volvulus*. Infestation with the former cause elephantiasis due to low grade inflammation which the parasite induces in the lymphatics and the latter causes subcutaneous nodules, looseness of the skin and blindness. *Wuchereria bancrofti* is transmitted by a female mosquito, usually of the *Culex* genus and onchocerca is transmitted by the fly, *Simulium damnosum*.

23.6 Mosquitoes transmit the following diseases:

1. Schistosomiasis
2. Leishmaniasis
3. Dengue
4. Yellow fever
5. Malaria

1. False
The mosquito plays no part in the life cycle of the schistosoma, the intermediate host of this parasite is a snail found in fresh water, see 23.4.

2. False
Leishmaniasis is a protozoal disease transmitted by the bite of the sandfly, *Phlebotomus papatasi*.

3. True
Dengue fever is a severe but usually short lived febrile illness which is caused by a toga virus transmitted by the mosquito *Aedes aegypti*.

4. True
Yellow fever is also caused by a toga virus transmitted by *Aedes aegypti*. Both the virus of dengue fever and yellow fever belong to the group collectively known as arthropod born virus, hence the generic name arbovirus.

5. True
Malaria is a protozoal disease transmitted by the female anopheles mosquito. The various protozoal species are *Plasmodium vivax*, *falciparum*, *malariae* and *ovale*. The most severe form of malaria is caused by *Pl. falciparum* which causes both cerebral malaria and blackwater fever. The latter is so named because of the haemoglobinuria which follows the severe intravascular haemolysis.

23.7 The following are mainly intracellular parasites:

1. *Echinococcus granulosus*
2. *Leishmania donovani*
3. *Trypanosoma gambiense*
4. *Plasmodium vivax*
5. *Toxoplasma gondii*

1. False

Echinococcus granulosus is a cestode (tapeworm) infestation which gives rise to hydatid disease. The dog is the intermediate host between sheep and man. In the latter the chief pathological lesion is the formation of hydatid cysts. These are most commonly found in the liver, lung, and brain, in descending order of frequency. The worms themselves are extracellular and infection develops when ova are accidentally eaten. These are shed in the faeces of the dogs which harbour the adult worm in the small intestine.

2. True

Leishmania donovani, a protozoon, is the causative agent of systemic leishmaniasis, kala-azar, a disease in which the protozoa are generally found within the macrophages in the amastigote form called the Leishman–Donovan bodies. These are particularly common in the bone marrow and spleen.

3. False

The trypanosomes, *T. gambiense* and *T. rhodesiense* are flagellated parasites which are found freely circulating in the blood. Both cause sleeping sickness in cattle and the human and are transmitted from man to man or from animals to man by the tsetse fly (*Glossina*).

4. True

Plasmodium vivax is one of a group of parasites of the genus *Plasmodium*. This particular species is responsible for benign tertian malaria. The diagnosis is confirmed by the examination of a blood smear when various forms of the life cycle including trophozoites, merozoites and schizonts can be seen within infected erythrocytes.

5. True

Toxoplasma gondii, the cause of toxoplasmosis, multiplies within the cytoplasm of the cells of the mono-nuclear phagocyte system causing the lymph nodes to enlarge and become packed with large cells which are probably macrophages. In severe cases cysts may form and in the brain necrotic nodules may be found which may calcify. Severe damage can also occur in the eye leading to choroidoretinitis and uveitis. The definitive host is the cat and infection occurs through faecal contamination of the human either by inhalation or ingestion. In the cat oocysts are discharged into the lumen from their site of development in the gastrointestinal membrane.

23.8 Autosomal dominant diseases which are important to surgeons include:

1. hereditary spherocytosis
2. haemophilia
3. Von Recklinghausen's disease
4. familial agammaglobulinaemia
5. mucoviscidosis

1. True
Congenital spherocytosis (spherocytic haemolytic anaemia) is due to the erythrocytes being more nearly spherical than normal. The result is a condition in which the life span of the erythrocytes is reduced. The abnormal cells are sequestrated in the spleen. Clinically, anaemia, intermittent jaundice and increasing splenomegaly occur.

2. False
Although haemophilia is a disease of considerable surgical importance it is rare, affecting only 6 per 100 000 of the population. It is normally inherited as a sex-linked recessive characteristic although sporadic cases do occur. The male exhibits the disease and the female acts as a carrier transmitting the disease to the next generation.

3. True
Von Recklinghausen's disease, otherwise known as neurofibromatosis, is associated with multiple nodules on the peripheral, and in some cases along the visceral branches of the sympathetic nerves. The disease is frequently associated with multiple pig-

mented patches of the skin, the café au lait spots. **The** various manifestations of this disease include:

(a) Multiple subcutaneous nodules associated with café au lait spots
(b) Dumb-bell tumours of the spinal nerves
(c) Acoustic nerve neuroma
(d) Elephantiasis neuromatosa
(e) Plexiform neuromata

4. False
Otherwise known as infantile sex-linked hypogammaglobulinaemia this condition may exist in the presence of normal cell mediated immunity. It is, however, inherited as an X-linked recessive.

5. False
This condition is inherited as an autosomal recessive. To the surgeon this condition presents with congenital intestinal obstruction, the muscular power of the intestine being insufficient to propel the viscid meconium. To the paediatrician milder forms of the condition present with failure of the affected infant to thrive and recurrent pulmonary infections.

23.9 Chromosome abnormalities may occur:

1. in Klinefelter's syndrome
2. following treatment with methotrexate
3. as a result of ionising radiation
4. in Down's syndrome
5. in Christmas disease

1. True
This is a condition occurring in males associated with an additional X chromosome, XXY. The clinical characteristics of the syndrome are the eunuchoid body structure, gynaecomastia and small underdeveloped testes.

2. False
Methotrexate does not directly affect the chromosomes.

3. True
Ionising radiation produces both 'sticky' chromosomes and breaks in the chromosomes, causing diffi-

culties in the separation of the chromatids at anaphase.

4. True
An extra chromosome instead of the normal pair at No. 21 chromosome is a feature of Down's syndrome (Mongolism).

5. False
Christmas disease is clinically similar to haemophilia. It is not, however, associated with any chromosomal abnormality.

23.10 Serum levels of HBsAg may be high in:

1. lepromatous leprosy
2. tuberculosis
3. Down's syndrome
4. heroin addicts
5. malignant melanoma

1. True
The titre of HBsAg antigen tends to be high in the inmates of institutions such as prisons and leprosaria. Since the majority of individuals suffering from lepromatous leprosy are found in leprosaria, it follows that a higher than normal incidence of HBsAg positivity occurs in these patients.

2. False
Since the treatment of tuberculosis no longer requires long term residence in sanatoria an increased incidence of HBsAg positivity in this condition does not occur.

3. True
A higher incidence of HBsAg than normal has been reported in Down's syndrome. The cause for this remains unknown and is particularly difficult to explain since these patients are not usually confined to institutions or particularly immunodeficient.

4. True
Heroin addicts have a high incidence of HBsAg positivity because of their use of contaminated syringes and needles.

5. False
Patients suffering from neoplastic diseases do not

appear to have an increased incidence of HBsAg positivity. They are, however, at risk if they require multiple transfusions or long stay residence in hospital.

23.11 The glycogen storage diseases are associated with the following enzyme defects:

1. Amylase
2. Glucose-6-phosphatase
3. Amylo, 1, 6-glycosidase
4. Glutamic oxaloacetic transaminase
5. Nucleotide adenophosphodehydrogenase

1. False
Amylase is the enzyme secreted by the exocrine portion of the pancreas and is responsible for the digestion of carbohydrate. In acute pancreatitis excessive quantities of this enzyme may be found in the blood enabling the diagnosis to be made.

2. True
Absence of this enzyme leads to von Gierke's disease (Type 1 glycogen storage disease). This disease develops in childhood and is associated with hepatomegaly and xanthomatosis.

3. True
A defect in this enzyme leads to a Type III glycogen storage disease, known eponymously as Ciris disease which resembles von Gierke's disease but is less severe.

4. False
Glutamic oxaloacetic transaminase is unrelated to glycogen storage diseases. It is an enzyme found in the liver, heart, kidneys and skeletal muscles concerned with transamination, i.e. the process whereby deamination of an amino acid is coupled with the amination of a ketoacid.

5. False
NADH dehydrogenase is an enzyme found in the brain. The energy status of any given area of the brain is most accurately expressed in terms of the ratio nucleotide adenophosphate (NAD^+) and NADH.

23.12 A vaccine:

1. contains one or more antigens
2. produces active immunity
3. contains one or more antibodies
4. stimulates polymorphonuclear leucocyte activity
5. can be administered orally

1. True
A vaccine contains antigenic material derived from one or more pathogenic organisms. These may be viral or bacterial and the organisms may be live, attenuated or dead.

2. True
Active immunity is produced following the administration of a vaccine by the stimulation of antibody production by the plasma cells which are themselves derived from B-lymphocytes.

3. False
Vaccines contain antigens. Immunisation against diptheica toxin may be produced with toxin–antitoxin floccules (TAF).

4. False
A vaccine has no effect on polymorphonuclear leucocyte activity.

5. True
Vaccines may be administered in a number of ways. The most common orally administered vaccine is the poliomyelitis vaccine introduced by Sabin which consists of living attenuated strains which have undergone mutation after passage through monkey-kidney cell cultures. The disadvantages associated with this type of vaccine are that the virus may not enter the cells of the intestinal tract and, therefore, no immunity develops and secondly, that the virus may undergo mutation in the alimentary tract reverting to a more virulent type which may then infect others.

23.13 Prostaglandins are:

1. formed from complement
2. vasodilators
3. involved in clotting

4. inhibited by azathioprine
5. inhibited by aspirin

1. False
The prostaglandins are derivatives of arachidonic acid which is present in every tissue of the body. However, the main source of this group of compounds is the platelets which contain enzymes capable of converting arachidonate into prostaglandins. Complement is an enzymatic system of serum proteins activated by antigen-antibody reactions.

2. True
Vasodilatation and increased capillary permeability are produced by PGE1 and PGE2, thus explaining the role of these compounds in acute inflammation. PGF2 protects the tissues from this action.

3. True
Prostaglandins are involved in clotting because a powerful platelet aggregator, thromboxane A2, is formed from prostaglandins G2 and H2. The enzymes involved are released when platelets become adherent to vessel walls.

4. False
Azathioprine does not inhibit the action of prostaglandins. It is, however, an immunosuppressive drug related to 6-mercaptopurine which is used in the treatment of diseases with an immunological basis including systemic lupus erythematosus, rheumatoid arthritis and Crohn's disease.

5. True
Aspirin inhibits the action of prostaglandins by the direct inhibition of their formation from the substrate arachidonic acid. This is thought to be the basis of its anti-inflammatory effect.